"A practical guide to unleashing our inner artist! Slom beautifully helps us step out of self-consciousness (and everything else that gets in the way) into awareness, connection, and self-expression."

>—**Jud Brewer, MD, PhD**, author of *The Craving Mind*, and director of research and innovation for the Mindfulness Center at Brown University

"This is a wonderful and wise book inviting us all to explore both our creativity and heart. Take a few moments to pause, feel into your body and mind, and experience its aliveness that seeds all possibility. *An Artful Path to Mindfulness* is filled with wisdom, kindness, and hope—that love and awareness will see us through and through."

>—**Bob Stahl, PhD**, coauthor of five books: *A Mindfulness-Based Stress Reduction Workbook*, *Living with Your Heart Wide Open*, *Calming the Rush of Panic*, *A Mindfulness-Based Stress Reduction Workbook for Anxiety*, and *MBSR Every Day*

"*An Artful Path to Mindfulness* offers step-by-step, clear, and practical techniques for understanding, absorbing, and learning mindfulness that allows us the experience of actually *being* mindful. There are many teachers of mindfulness, but none before offered such detailed ways to understand the steps that lead us to mindfulness. In my opinion, the beauty of this book rests in the practicality of its content which is both concrete and softly esoteric, allowing us to absorb the tools for understanding and 'owning' the steps to mindful inner peace. Thank you, Janet, for the gift you have given to all of us."

>—**Rabbi Roger Ross**, chair of New Vision Interspiritual Seminary; executive director of the Rabbinical Seminary International; United Nations (UN) representative of the NGO, United Religions Initiative; and cochair of the Committee on Spirituality, Values, and Global Concerns at the UN

"Enter this book with an open mind and let Janet Slom guide you on the path of creativity. The joys of absorption, fearlessness, and discovery await. Give yourself enough time, take patience with you—and the rewards will be life-changing."

>—**Amy Gross**, former editor in chief of *O, The Oprah Magazine*; and mindfulness-based stress reduction (MBSR) teacher

"*An Artful Path to Mindfulness*—based on activities from MBSR—evokes innate, spacious awareness while cultivating curiosity, creativity, and freedom. Janet Slom wholeheartedly extends an invitation to play at the edges of not knowing, and discovery of natural rhythms through each exploration with mindful art encounters. The workbook offers the structure and inspiration to draw from deep inner resources, seeing clearly, and resting in the unfolding of intimacy and interconnection with self, others, and the natural world."

>—**Florence Meleo-Meyer, MS, MA, LMFT**, program director of global relations and professional education for the Mindfulness Center at Brown University

"Janet Slom invites the reader to consider drawing, not as an object but as a process—a personal journey. Through a series of practical exercises, she avoids teaching drawing as the acquisition of empty skills. Instead, she encourages the reader to consider drawing as a visual process that can effectively explore the space of thought and feeling. Janet Slom's book, *An Artful Path to Mindfulness*, is ambitious; she believes if the act of drawing is fully embraced as a 'mindful' vehicle for rigorous self-discovery, not only will the resulting drawings be more meaningful and deeply compelling, they may change your life."

—**Power Boothe**, professor of painting in the Hartford Art School at the University of Hartford

"This is a thinking-out-of-the box program author Janet Slom calls mindfulness-based self-expression, or MSBE. She encourages creativity, various art exercises, and entertaining possibilities we haven't dared to. Instead of living reactively, Slom urges we engage life as it is to experience our true selves and live joyfully."

—**Sharon Salzberg**, author of *Real Happiness* and *Lovingkindness*

"Create, preserve, destroy in order to recreate freshly! Through an ingenious, inventive, and mature reimagining of the MBSR curriculum, Janet draws us lovingly into the dance of 'making marks.' Holding firmly to the essence of mindfulness, this book is a point of light shining forth from the depths of Janet's heart and the brilliance of her art."

—**Saki F. Santorelli, EDD, MA**, educator, meditation teacher, writer, and pioneer in integrating meditation and mindfulness into medicine, health care, and the broader society; former executive director of the Center for Mindfulness in Medicine, Health Care, and Society; director of the internationally acclaimed Stress Reduction Clinic; and professor of medicine at the University of Massachusetts Medical School

"MBSE is an invaluable and innovative practice for accessing our unique creative flow, and applying it to our lives. Whether making a mark on canvas or in the world, mindfulness and creativity are essential resources. Janet Slom is an inspiring and compassionate guide who offers an easy-to-follow methodology; even after just a few exercises, MBSE effectively replenishes and enriches us. This book is an invitation to a dynamic exploration of self-discovery and self-expression."

—**Jeff Elster**, eco entrepreneur and artist who has been studying and practicing meditation in the US and India for more than thirty years

"In a world where there is much being written about mindfulness, it is refreshing to discover a novel and accessible book which retains fidelity to the core tenets of both contemporary mindfulness and its dharmic roots, while skilfully synthesising these practices with creative and artistic forms that will nourish, heal, and reveal in equal measure."

—**Simon Whitesman, MD**, medical psychotherapist in private practice in Cape Town, South Africa; and director of the Institute for Mindfulness South Africa, and postgraduate training in mindfulness-based interventions at Stellenbosch University

"In her outstanding book, Janet Slom invites us to set aside preconceived notions, assumptions, beliefs, and assessments, to fully engage the present moment with an open mind and heart. As a participant in her workshops, I have experienced the positive and enduring impact of her unique approach to stress reduction through exploring creativity and presenting our true selves to the world. Thankfully, now, many more people can access her theories and approaches in this workbook. Janet combines the multiple roles of teacher, artist, poet, and dancer to guide readers through their personalized ninety-day program toward a healthy life. As a psychologist assisting others in their own challenging journeys, I look forward to incorporating this timely book into my work."

—**Dale Atkins, PhD**, practicing psychologist, lecturer, media commentator, and author of seven books, including *The Kindness Advantage*; *Sanity Savers*; *Wedding Sanity Savers*; *I'm OK, You're My Parents*; *From the Heart*; and *Sisters*

"Every mining expedition begins in the dark. We don't know what riches are hidden in the depths, yet the process demands that we move into the unknown. Janet's expert guidance supports a path of soulful discovery towards self-expression, creativity, and self-knowing. Skillfully integrating practices of mindful awareness with various means of artistic expression in original and deeply embodied ways, Janet's methods include meditations, reflections, experiments, and mindful art encounters. Through this progression, we can touch jewels of courage and tenderness, experience play and wonder, and illumine freedom in forgotten places. The light of awareness is the perfect beacon to penetrate layers of old judgments and limitations. The motherlode, we discover, is the journey itself—priceless and beyond compare."

—**Lynn Koerbel, MPH**, assistant director of MBSR teacher education and curricular development at the Mindfulness Center at Brown University, and coauthor of A *Mindfulness-Based Stress Reduction Workbook for Anxiety*

"If as Paul Cezanne said, 'we live in a rainbow of chaos,' encountering Janet Slom within this book is like bumping into an iron angel who hoists Cezanne's rainbow into the sky with bold encouragement and unconditional acceptance. There's beauty in chaos, and vast relief when we let go of urges to fix or make it better. Janet's wholehearted fearlessness to uplift and inspire new perceptions of our magical, mysterious, chaotic, catastrophic, beautiful, brief consciousness known as human life is both startling and radical. Her life's work and passion, skillfully unveiled within the practices of MBSE, roots deep into our historic landscape of stress and suffering. By undoing the so-called self-image, shifting us into being and seeing from the heart, 'artfulness' invites us to be just as we are, wildly free and alive. The courage to represent our perfectly imperfect, flawed yet fabulous, unadulterated creativity as genuine expressions of love and self-acceptance requires a radical re-visioning of what we have imagined ourselves and art to be. Janet's bold guidance encourages us to dust away constructed identities that separate art from invisibility and 'self' from 'other,' inspiring us to awaken together a larger, more joyful state of creative awareness. Enjoy!"

—**Debra Annane, MA, MPH, RYT**, mindfulness practitioner, facilitator, and researcher

AN *Artful* PATH
TO
MINDFULNESS

MBSR-BASED ACTIVITIES for
USING CREATIVITY TO
REDUCE STRESS & EMBRACE
THE PRESENT MOMENT

JANET SLOM, MFA

New Harbinger Publications, Inc.

Publisher's Note

This publication is designed to provide accurate and authoritative information in regard to the subject matter covered. It is sold with the understanding that the publisher is not engaged in rendering psychological, financial, legal, or other professional services. If expert assistance or counseling is needed, the services of a competent professional should be sought.

Distributed in Canada by Raincoast Books

Copyright © 2020 by Janet Slom
               New Harbinger Publications, Inc.
               5674 Shattuck Avenue
               Oakland, CA 94609
               www.newharbinger.com

Cover design by Sara Christian

Interior design by Michele Waters-Kermes

Acquired by Elizabeth Hollis Hansen

All Rights Reserved

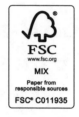 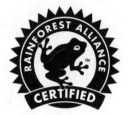

FSC
www.fsc.org
MIX
Paper from
responsible sources
FSC® C011935

Library of Congress Cataloging-in-Publication Data on file

Printed in the United States of America

22   21   20

10   9   8   7   6   5   4   3   2   1   First Printing

Contents

Foreword   v

Introduction: Welcome to the Artful Path   1

Week 1   Who Am I?   11
Nine Dots   18
Mindful Art Encounter #1: Who Am I?   20
Mindful Art Encounter #2: Finding Your Personal Mark   22
Mindful Art Encounter #3: Exploring Your Personal Mark   24
Mindful Art Encounter #4: Freedom of Self-Expression   26
Mindful Art Encounter #5: Body Scan Self-Portrait   28

Week 2   Opening to Your Reality   35
Mindful Eating   41
Mindful Art Encounter #6: Conversation Drawing with Self   44
Mindful Art Encounter #7: Letting Go   47
Mindful Art Encounter #8: Rebuilding, Collage Part 1   49
Mindful Art Encounter #9: Opening to Your Reality   50

Week 3   Being Present   55
Mindful Art Encounter #10: Taking Off the Mask   60
Mindful Art Encounter #11: Accepting   65
Mindful Art Encounter #12: Seeing Clearly   67
Mindful Art Encounter #13: Self-Portrait: Seeing Things as They Are   69

Week 4   Playing   73
Mindful Art Encounter #14: Surprise and Play   77
Mindful Art Encounter #15: The Ugly Drawing   79
Mindful Art Encounter #16: Destruction and Tearing Apart   82
Mindful Art Encounter #17: Rebuilding, Collage Part 2   84

Week 5   Accepting Wholeness   89
    Mindful Art Encounter #18: Exploring Yin and Yang   93
    Mindful Art Encounter #19: Exploring Judgment   97
    Mindful Art Encounter #20: Exploring Acceptance   99
    Mindful Art Encounter #21: Embracing Yin and Yang   101

Week 6   Communicating   105
    Mindful Art Encounter #22: Listening Enemy or Friend?   112
    Mindful Art Encounter #23: Drawing and Collaging with Words   115
    Mindful Art Encounter #24: Engaged Listening   118
    Mindful Art Encounter #25: Listening to Your Whispers   120
    Mindful Art Encounter #26: Conversation Drawing with a Partner   123

Week 7   A Retreat of Silence, Simplicity, and Solitude   129

Week 8   Going Deeper and Wider   135
    Mindful Art Encounter #27: Being the Wind   139
    Mindful Art Encounter #28: Being the Ocean   140
    Mindful Art Encounter #29: Being the River   143
    Mindful Art Encounter #30: Being the Sky   144
    Mindful Art Encounter #31: Being a Tree   145
    Mindful Art Encounter #32: Conversation Drawing with Community   146

Week 9   Who Am I Now?   153
    Mindful Art Encounter #33: Mandala: The Heart of Being   157
    Mindful Art Encounter #34: Planting Seeds, Growing Flowers   160
    Mindful Art Encounter #35: Who Am I Now?   162

Conclusion: Celebrating Each Moment: Mindfulness for the Rest of Your Life   167

Acknowledgments   171

Practice Logs   173

More Mindfulness Resources   183

References   191

Foreword

Janet Slom is an artist. And art is what we are concerned with here, whether it be in the cultivation of meditative awareness or in painting, sculpture, collage, dance, music, poetry, or any other form of human expression.

What Janet is offering us with this participatory engagement she calls *mindfulness-based self-expression* is itself an exquisite art form: the art of living life as if it really mattered. And what you may not know but may have very much intuited in reaching for this book in the first place, is that it does matter.... in more ways than you might think. In fact, I would say that it matters in more ways than you or any of us *can* think—because thinking is not always all that it is cracked up to be. And even at its best and most rigorous and authentic, thinking is only one of a range of multiple intelligences we are gifted with from birth—each of us carrying our own unique mix of elements that ultimately drive the particular ways in which our creative and imaginative impulses might reveal themselves and be expressed—if we are lucky enough. And lucky we are to be a recipient of this invitation. For one of Janet's many gifts is her ability to bring to life the art of mindfulness, both as a disciplined meditation practice and as a way of being. Mindfulness-based self-expression (MBSE), an offshoot of MBSR (mindfulness-based stress reduction), skillfully taps into our innate creativity, imagination, and capacity for discernment, as well as, in the end, our ability to love and fully inhabit the life that is ours to live.

The curriculum offered here is particularly meaningful to me because my mother was a painter her whole adult life, right up through age 101. In looking back daily over her innumerable sketchbooks in her last decades—for her a form of meditation she engaged in for many hours a day once she no longer could mobilize the energy and materials for painting on a regular basis—she would often criticize her work (gently and with a sense of humor) for not being "bold enough." She didn't shy away from reworking those sketches even forty or fifty years later, to take risks she somehow didn't dare take when she was younger and see what would happen. Growing up with her, I came to see a bit through her eyes because she was so passionate and vocal about seeing and making art. She saw and pointed out things that many of us never notice: reflections in windows, windshields, glass doors, and glass buildings, which we ordinarily tune out; the play of color and shadow in different lights; the emotional depths of each human face; the rich variability of body types and postures—all were captured by her eye and hand. They were essential elements of her universe, and sources of endless delight. She worshiped Monet, and I sometimes felt as if, in seeing through her eyes, I was seeing through his.

Janet is also a painter, and for many years, the walls of the Center for Mindfulness at UMass were graced with her work on loan. Her canvases, many quite large, lit up the building and the lives of all who entered the space.

Reflecting back in time for a moment, the Paleolithic cave paintings from circa 20,000 years ago at Lascaux in France and Altamira in Spain, and the more recent hand prints and other petroglyphs on the walls of canyons and caves in the Southwest of North America, are evidence that artistic representation is one of humankind's earliest and most long-enduring forms of cultural expression. They are also evidence of sophisticated technologies developed independently in many different locales from Paleolithic through Neolithic times, whether what was expressed was worked with paint, ink, pigments, or dyes. Somehow, the materials used and the images and narratives they captured astonishingly survived unimaginable weather conditions and exposure for millennia. They also capture with remarkable artistry and aliveness the forms of all kinds of animals and plants, presumably meaningful representations of the painters' community's place in the universe.

All these expressions are evidence of the deeply rooted impulse for human beings and societies to *leave their mark* and express meanings we can often only guess at. But what comes to mind are belonging, connectivity, dependency on other life forms, community, shared narratives, meaning, and mystery. Similar self-expressions manifested in unique ways and styles throughout human history in virtually all cultures, whether it be Abyssinian, Persian, Egyptian, Greek, Chinese, Japanese, European, Mayan, Inuit, Australian Aboriginal, Maori, African, to name just a few, and continue to do so right to this very day. And not just in representational forms: equally profound expressions are found of course in abstract art, music, poetry, dance, photography, as well as in the sciences and scholarly pursuits of all kinds. Artistic expression is woven into our DNA.

Among the most creative and revealing exercises in this book are those moments, and there are many, when we are invited to leave *our mark*, or many of them, and thereby enjoy a spontaneity in doing so that reveals its own expressions of emotion, intelligence, and meaning, transcending our all-too-frequently-merely-habitual cognitions. And then go further, and not be attached to whatever we produced, or to notice if we are. In other words, to recognize the impermanent and non-self nature of what has emerged as we repurpose it on purpose for the next expression of what might reveal itself.

As Janet's curriculum makes amply clear, there are any number of creative and artistic pathways open to us. Life itself is an art form, or can be. Meditation is too. Mindfulness meditation is nothing other than the art of conscious embodied living. As Henry David Thoreau put it in Walden, "To affect the quality of the day, that is the highest of arts."

Not only is meditation an art form. Ultimately it is at one and the same time a love affair with the magic and power to be discovered, uncovered, recovered, or revealed in silence; in stillness; in awareness; and in embodied action for the sake of others and the world. These are no less art forms themselves, profound forms of self-expression realized.

That said, what we mean by "the self" is itself brought into focus and into question in the meditative arts. Who in fact is the artist? Who is the meditator? Who is breathing? What or who is seeing? Who am

I, when you come right down to it? Where do I belong? Who are we? Where do I fit in to the larger picture? And what would best express what is in my heart? In other words, how can I leave my mark and make a difference? And how can I appreciate the marks of others in my circle of interconnected being and belong? This is the heart of the curriculum unfolded within these pages. It is also the heart of the motivation to engage in the adventure of being alive in this era—not that different and hardly less mysterious, for all the distance we have come, than it must have been in ancient times when we lived in caves and marveled at the night sky as we looked out rather than up, and at the unimaginable power of nature.

Such questions as those posed in the paragraph above are not so much to be answered as to be reflected upon and inquired into. They point to mysteries that call out for a personal embodied awake encounter and for an authentic momentary response, which often manifests as art, whether on the wall of a cave or canyon then, or on a piece of paper now, or in an uncontrived natural awareness of the carriage of the body while sitting, walking, hearing, speaking, dancing, loving, whatever the moment invites out of us.

Challenging as the adventure of discovering and embodying our unique potential is, fortunately Janet is here to guide us in this adventure and investigation of what may be deepest and best in ourselves, and most important to express and possibly share. There are an infinite number of doors into the universe of a life lived fully and well. And there are also an infinite number of doors into the cultivation of mindfulness and heartfulness. It is life itself and how we live it that is the ultimate art form and the real meditation practice, no matter what unique form it may take in different moments once we are willing to wake up a bit more, come to our senses, see with eyes of wholeness, and befriend our own capacity for full awareness and not-knowing, nothing less than a willingness to be open and to be surprised.

In that sense, this book is a huge and empty canvas. Or maybe it is your life that is the empty canvas in this or any moment. We can't know for sure until we say "yes" to the invitation to engage and then… actually engage, giving ourselves over to Janet's expert and compassionate guidance and to "the curriculum" of life itself and what it calls out of us. In the end, I hope you find the art of mindfulness both healing and freeing, as so many others have.

May this workbook and its carefully calibrated curriculum prove to be a portal for you into a universe of ongoing self-expression that transcends any limited or limiting conceptualizations of who you are. And may it illuminate the many ways in which you can gift your creativity and genius to the world, and to yourself.

I wish you all the best with this adventure of a lifetime.

—Jon Kabat-Zinn
October 20, 2019
Northampton, MA

Welcome to the Artful Path

In today's rush, we all think too much, seek too much, want too much, and forget about the joy of just being.

—Eckhart Tolle, *A New Earth*

Years ago, a man came to my studio for his private lesson. He was a highly successful entrepreneur who had, in every material sense, created a model life. As soon as I answered the door, he expressed skepticism about the lessons, wondering if it would be a waste of time.

"How do you feel about embarking on this new experience?" I asked him.

After a few seconds, Sam replied, "I have no idea how I feel." He had been so busy traveling, negotiating, and reaching his goals that he was numb. "I know that success is not bringing me happiness," he said. Though everyone around him looked up to him and regarded him as successful, inside he felt like a failure. I could sense he had lost his connection to his intuition.

I invited him to come into the studio and leave expectations outside the door. We began with a mark-making exercise. Sam expressed frustration and impatience. For the first time in a while, he wasn't an expert at what he was doing. He remained skeptical about the process.

Over the next two weeks we began to explore the creative process together, introducing mindfulness practice, journaling, yoga, and creative art exercises. During our third meeting, I witnessed one of the most dramatic shifts in my years of teaching. Tears rolled down Sam's cheeks as he worked through one of the art exercises, and his creative energy began to flow. I could see his joy in the moment. The tentative marks of previous weeks became strong, direct, and playful. He became curious and engaged. He was in the process of play. Rather than simply considering a concept, he was feeling firsthand the emotions and sensations of *experience*.

After that day, Sam understood the difference between direct experience and the concept of *present-moment awareness*. Rather than grasping for a future or dwelling on the past, as he had been, he began to immerse himself in and feel moments of presence. He started making choices that allowed time for practice, play, and stepping outside the fast track to another now. Empowered and energized, he continued exploring art, movement, and mindfulness, and his direct experience flowed into other areas of his life.

Many of us may recognize aspects of ourselves in Sam's story. When you look at your life, do you feel it is working just the way it is? Or do you long for meaning, connection, love, and well-being? Do you feel overwhelmed, anxious, stressed, debilitated by pain, depression, or disease? Are you stuck in whatever challenge or suffering you may be experiencing? Have you been numbing through addictions to food, drink, your phone, the Internet, being busy, sex, work, pushing, striving, competing, or whatever it is that offers escape? So many of us are stuck in the groove of habitual pushing away, numbly living reactively rather than proactively, and feeling exhausted.

I have worked with many successful people who are unhappy. They conform to societal expectations, following instructions from others about how they are supposed to be. Like many of us, they are outer-focused, looking for answers "out there": in books and courses, in the opinions of leaders, family, teachers, and peers. Meanwhile, they have no idea of who they are.

There is, however, a different way. It starts with a journey inward—of self-exploration, of looking at things as they are, and committing to being in your life as if it truly matters, as if this is the most important work you can do. It requires the awareness that arises with no longer going through your days on automatic pilot. This is what I call an *artful path*. It's a journey to discovering joy in presence. Because joy can only be felt in the present moment, it requires slowing down and tuning in to direct experience, engaging and immersing in the present moment, alert, aware, awake, and being with things as they are.

Who are you in your innermost self now? What brings you joy? What is meaningful to you? This is the work, and it requires self-compassion, commitment, and intention, but nothing can be more important. It is only once you blossom from your core, invoking creativity and engaging creative energy and self-compassion, that you can in turn love others and together we can enjoy an interdependent, interconnected, inclusive way of being in this world.

LIVING MINDFULLY ON AN ARTFUL PATH

The only place to experience life fully is in the present moment. The past has already gone, and dwelling on it often leads to regrets, would-haves, should-haves, could-haves, memories of liking or disliking, and longings for more of what we remember liking and less of what we disliked. This process of past recollection keeps us from *experience*, which can only be felt in the present. Thinking about the past robs us of the precious now. On the other end, the future has not yet arrived. Focusing exclusively on the future—whether planning, hoping, anticipating, longing, worrying, or fearing the unknown—can cause us to lose touch with life living through us now, again taking us away from experiencing life in each moment.

This ability to be aware, awake to life in the present moment, with acceptance, and self-compassion, without judgment or trying to change anything, is known as "mindfulness." *Practicing* mindfulness includes noticing when we have thoughts about the past or future and directing our awareness back to the present moment experiences of seeing, hearing, smelling, tasting, touching, and sensing sensations in the body and emotions and thoughts in this moment.

How do we begin living mindfully? Becoming aware of body sensations, emotions, thoughts, and our senses as well as the visual language of art are ways to practice mindfulness—practices that are covered within these pages. *An Artful Path to Mindfulness* leads you through a nine-week program called "Mindfulness-Based Self-Expression," or MBSE, designed to awaken insight, cultivate mindfulness and self-compassion, and nurture creativity. Inspired by Jon Kabat-Zinn's classic mindfulness-based stress reduction (MBSR) program, MBSE combines traditional mindfulness practices with art encounters to help you direct your awareness to the present moment.

As we immerse ourselves in art exercises, we playfully adventure, deepening our connection to experience. We are becoming more alive in each moment. In fact, creativity is one of the keys to living a meaningful and fulfilling life. When our creative juices are flowing, we have the capacity to create, resolve, and respond with ease. We build resilience and trust, take risks, feel curious, and engage in play. When our creative impulse is blocked, on the other hand, we feel limited in our essence, ideas, solutions, and effectiveness. We become stuck in old habits, reactivity, and fear.

We are born with the ability to express and communicate through verbal, visual, musical, and physical languages. In today's Western culture, however, verbal language—thinking and concepts—tend to drown out the languages of the body (such as hearing, tasting, and feeling emotions and sensations). MBSE uses simple visual art exercises that awaken the creativity residing inside each of us. As we tap into the language of inner knowing, we stop listening to the judgmental voice within or from others. We connect with our innate being—our humanity—and with that which brings us joy.

Healing through art is an ancient practice rooted in many traditions, from the pre-Columbian Mayan to the Egyptian, African, and Indian. These cultures used drawing, painting, and sculpture as vehicles for telling stories, recording histories, sharing ideas, and expressing connections to land and ocean, nature and animals.

Is MBSE only for artists? Absolutely not! No artistic skill or experience is needed. All you need is this book, a pen or pencil, a separate journal or notebook, and a few (mostly basic) art supplies—and the time and willingness to get started. Just dive in and stay open to the possibilities of expressing your life visually.

As you work through the Mindfulness-Based Self-Expression program in this book, you'll practice, again and again, bringing awareness to:

- being in the present moment

- breathing and inhabiting your body

- observing your thoughts

- differentiating between thoughts, emotions, and sensations

- becoming aware of your habitual tendencies, with kindness and curiosity

- trusting the process of "not knowing" and rediscovering "beginner's mind"

- releasing control of things needing to be a certain way

- accepting that mistakes are creative opportunities, in both art and life

- practicing letting go and trusting the possibility of a new creation

- responding with care and attention, rather than reacting out of habit

- expanding your awareness and experiencing the moment more fully

- staying open to vulnerability and whatever arises

- communicating, both with yourself and others in an improvisational and fresh way

- being present when listening/speaking

- opening pathways to your unique creative essence

- simply being present to all that you are experiencing

- being kind

- nurturing yourself with compassion

There is no goal for this program. Also note that it is not art therapy. Rather, it is a journey to befriend and express yourself—a path that begins with one breath, one step, one mark on paper, a lifelong practice to begin again in each moment.

MY STORY

My journey with MBSE started on a flower farm in South Africa when I was four years old.

My family's flower farm was called Shamballa (common human goodness). From the very beginning, I was surrounded by both beauty and a keen awareness of humanity's immense suffering. In addition to being a farm for gladioli and carnations, Shamballa had been created by my father as a learning center for Eastern philosophy. A verandah stretched the entire length of our farmhouse, with four majestic plane trees forming a canopy above. As the wind created music in the leaves, I would sit on the verandah with my father, learning about breathing and meditation.

My father would instruct me to close my eyes and feel the sensations of my breath in my body. I would feel my belly rise on the in-breath and return on the out-breath, learning to bring attention to the breath without trying to change it in any way. My father would gently ask me whether the breath coming into the body was longer than the breath leaving. As we exhaled, we would visualize sending messages of loving kindness to everything around us on the farm: the flowers, the trees, the animals, the river, our family, and friends, taking in their love and goodness as we inhaled.

My father would then invite me to listen to the songs of the birds. We'd listen quietly for fifteen minutes. When we opened our eyes, we'd remain silent for a while and then talk about the experience.

One time, I reached for crayons next to me and began drawing the feelings and colors of listening and speaking. My father quietly looked at the drawing without judging or trying to interpret it. He encouraged me to speak about the drawing process, its messages, and how the songs of the birds felt. I remember feeling happy for our quiet time together. We were sharing silence and stillness, listening and speaking, curiosity, wonder, and delight. I felt a deep sense of peace and gratitude.

We would close our eyes again, this time bringing our attention to the leaves rustling in the breeze. I could feel the wind on my cheeks and the sensation of inhabiting the leaves' music. The leaves were dancing in the wind, and everything danced together.

When I was six years old, all of the buds on our farm wilted. This was a cause for deep concern for my parents. The flowers were to be exported to England and were our only source of income. Mr. Brown flew out from London to test the soil. He walked the property, and after a long while, returned to the verandah. The soil had a rare and irreversible disease, he said. There was nothing that could be done. My parents would have to close the farm. My father lowered his head in silence, and Mr. Brown left. My mother began to sob uncontrollably. We had no money, no savings. Everything had been put into the land.

My father called my four-year-old brother, Richard, and me onto the verandah. I'd never seen my mother so distressed, and my father looked deeply sad. My brother and I held onto each other in fear.

To our surprise, my father looked up and told me to go put on my favorite party dress, the white one with the pink bow. He told Richard to dress in his khaki shorts and white shirt. He asked my mother to dry her tears and put on her pink suit, the one with the pearl buttons that she had not worn for such a long time. When we came back to the verandah in our special outfits, my father announced that we were going to Lambada for dinner. This was a fancy restaurant in the village; we had been there only once before.

As we sat down at the restaurant, my father asked us to all join hands. He looked silently into each of our eyes for a moment, and then we each did the same, going around the circle taking in each other's presence. We were filled with love and fear and sadness, not understanding what this was about.

My father began to speak in a soft voice. This was a very important moment in our lives, he said, one that we should always remember. "We have just lost our livelihood. You, too, will have many difficult moments of struggle, challenge, and loss. That is life. You will have gains and losses. We must remember to celebrate our losses as well as our gains. I do not know what we will do. I do not have a plan at this moment. I do know that we will take a moment to be still and be quiet. We will reinvent ourselves, and we will learn from this experience," he said.

We all hugged each other. Love would guide us. We would find a way. We breathed into the moment, feeling loss, sadness, fear, and worry—but also faith that we would be okay. The loving support for one another gave us strength as we adventured into our new lives, not knowing what the next moment would be.

As I felt all of the strong emotions in this experience, I found a place of acceptance and peace. Emotions and sensations surged through my body, changing from moment to moment. Looking back, I realize that the hours of meditation on the verandah, and the breathing awareness exercises that my father had taught me, helped me to navigate the bumps in the road.

Soon after this evening, my nursery school teacher, Mrs. Penny, noticed my sadness and gave me a few sheets of paper. She asked me to draw how I felt. She kneeled down and put her face close to mine. I looked into her eyes and saw that she understood my broken heart. She was present, kindly guiding me. It was a precious and transformative milestone that would shape my journey forever. I drew into my sadness, expressing it in lines, shapes, and forms. The hand holding the crayon was a lifeline from my heart, saying: *Trust...it will change.* And, eventually, it did.

As I grew up, my dedication and commitment to these practices deepened. I developed exercises to explore and investigate my way out of trouble, ways to unblock my feelings and mental clarity during intense challenges and loss so as to be in my life fully. I began teaching these exercises at a community center, and the classes grew, with students ranging from children to adults from all walks of life. The program evolved out of a lifetime of learning from many traditions and teachers—from my father on our verandah to the Dalai Lama, Jon Kabat-Zinn, Sharon Salzberg, Pema Chödrön, Eckhart Tolle, Thich Nhat Hanh, Krishna Murti, Alice Baily, gurus from India, yoga masters, Chögyam Trungpa Rinpoche's *Shambhala: The Sacred Path of the Warrior*, the Bhagavad Gita, and the Old and New Testaments—and became deeply intertwined with my work as an artist, dancer, yoga teacher, interfaith minister, and spiritual counselor.

In 2003, I completed Jon Kabat-Zinn's mindfulness-based stress reduction (MBSR) program. It seemed only natural to blend the teachings I had already been sharing for thirty years with Jon's brilliant MBSR curriculum, and thus mindfulness based self-expression was born. I have since taught MBSE to thousands of participants around the world and have seen the transformative results regardless of age, gender, religion, education, ethnicity, profession, or material status. Students have called the course "energizing," "an invaluable experience," and "a lifetime experience that I will forever carry with me."

WHY DRAW?

As you follow the MBSE journey, you may notice that many of the activities involve drawing. Why drawing? And what does it have to do with mindfulness?

Drawing is a visual expression innate to all human beings. Just as words form a language, lines, shapes, forms, and marks are the vocabulary of drawing. These marks are unique for each of us, just like our handwriting. The way we arrange and compose lines, shapes, forms, and gestures is a visual conversation. Through drawing, we can tell stories, express emotions, reveal insights, and inspire ourselves (and others). Through drawing, we access the invisible, bringing our inner and outer worlds together. Drawing can be a doorway to expression, understanding, and healing.

MBSE focuses on abstract drawing and requires no technical ability—only the courage to venture into mark-making in a way that feels intuitive, natural, and new. It's less about the *product* than it is about the *process*. Each time you face a blank page it requires becoming curious, being present, leaving judgment behind, and taking risks.

The process of abstract drawing is alive, requiring you to make choices in each moment that are spontaneous. There are no rules. Each of us experiences the world differently, and as you play with lines, marks, shapes, patterns, and texture without conforming to or copying others, you speak a language of self-expression that is genuine, accessing parts of yourself that may be hidden. The results are usually surprising. Each drawing becomes a visual interpretation of your moment-to-moment journey, of your unique expression. It is an act of affirming your presence in the world.

Approached in this way, drawing becomes a tool to access your true nature and to practice being awake and aware. It helps you build your ability to take risks, see options, choose how to respond, engage with play and curiosity, and feel into each moment.

When I was eight years old, I had a teacher who insisted that we copy objects exactly. Some of my classmates were experts in copying. I, on the other hand, was always inspired to *interpret* what I saw rather than make a representational drawing. Where copying felt restrictive, my intuitive way of drawing was like a dance that flowed onto the page, filled with ease and joy.

My teacher was not impressed. Her harsh judgments—and praise of more compliant students who echoed her way of expression—led me to feel that I wasn't good enough to be an artist. Deeply saddened, I stopped painting.

Years later I found my way back to drawing, playing with lines, shapes and forms, texture, composition, and design, enjoying the process rather than the product or goal. It was a way for me to explore the world and make sense of my life. Everything seemed more colorful, more alive, and clearer as I drew into and explored my questions, my sadness, and my joy. I befriended all of my experiences—even the challenging and dark ones, drawing into and through the darkness with kindness and understanding.

Drawing does not have to represent the outer world. It does not have to be about objects. It can be whatever you want it to be. You are the guide of your own expression. Your only responsibility is to explore, experiment, and live from your core values and intention—and in so doing, connect with your genuine creative voice and share your unique way with the world.

If you feel reluctant to try this medium of expression, what's holding you back? Is it thoughts such as *I am not creative; It won't turn out well;* or *It's a waste of time?*

Fear has a way of keeping us stuck in familiar ways. Facing a blank piece of paper is a metaphor for beginning again and not holding onto old habits. It requires being with fear and working with it, rather than denying it, pushing it away, or numbing it. As we begin each new drawing with one fresh mark, letting go of past drawings, we are training ourselves to live in the present without hanging onto the past. We are learning to call upon our intuition and inspiration to follow with the next mark, building a visual record—or, indeed, a life—made of marks and gestures that are immediate and true in each moment.

As you explore the drawing exercises in this book, be kind to yourself. Try not to judge, compare, or evaluate. Are you speaking to yourself with encouragement, being your own best friend? If you speak harshly to yourself, pause, say you are sorry, and give yourself an internal hug. *I'm sorry. Please forgive me. Thank you for coming home to your heart of kindness and self-compassion.* Invite in the voice of encouragement and befriending.

THE JOURNEY OF MINDFULNESS-BASED SELF-EXPRESSION

Mindfulness-Based Self-Expression is a practice and a path. It's a doorway into your heart, a way of tapping into the core of your uniqueness and then celebrating who you are by living in a direct, engaged, wise, and creative way. We all feel loss and judgment, fear and anxiety, regret and worry. We all long for happiness, peace, understanding, and love. All of us have times of darkness and doubt. You are not alone. Whether or not you decide to share your journey with others, realizing this can help you feel communion with the rest of humanity.

The nine-week structure is one I have honed over my years of teaching MBSE in scores of group settings. It's a rich and well-developed program that builds week by week, with the transformations that naturally occur with practice, in the tradition of the ground-breaking mindfulness-based stress reduction (MBSR) program developed by Jon Kabat-Zinn and his colleagues at the University of Massachusetts Medical School.

The MBSE program requires practice, intention, commitment, and dedication to being mindful in your life.

Following the program, you will practice mindful creativity each week in two ways:

- through building a daily practice of body-centered exercises, including the body scan, gentle stretching yoga, sitting meditation, walking meditation, and loving-kindness meditation; and

- through choosing from a group of Mindful Art Encounters through which you will explore your creative process of self-expression.

There is no single right way or wrong way to do Mindfulness-Based Self Expression—there is only your way. *You* are the ultimate guide of your own learning and practice.

PRACTICING WITH THIS WORKBOOK

This workbook is designed to be encountered in several ways, and how you use it is up to you. It can be used as a guide to the full nine-week MBSE program, as an inspiration for and record of your self-exploration, as a resource for you to revisit over time—or all of these. To support your work with the materials in this book, a host of materials are available for download from the book's website, http://www.new harbinger.com/44932, including text and audio instructions of all the meditation exercises, PDF versions of some of the workbook exercises that you may want to do again, and printable worksheets.

Each chapter in this workbook is designed to be completed in a week, blending self-exploration, self-expression, and body-centered mindfulness practices. I encourage you to make your way through the workbook in order, one chapter per week. Many concepts and practices inform and build upon each other, and there is real benefit to be had in working through the full nine-week program in order. If you do this,

I encourage you to take at least a full week for each chapter, to give your body and mind time and space to take in the experience.

That being said, take from this program and these practices just exactly what you happen to need. Treat this MBSE workbook as a true friend offering nonjudgmental messages and insights to inform your path; ways for you to explore, experience, and connect to your deepest knowing; and a gentle invitation to step up and do the work necessary for a fulfilling and meaningful life. As you work through the book, feel free to play, tear, mark, and take risks. This is a container to store and keep safe your experience, recording your curiosity, vulnerability, resilience, strength, and creativity as you show up for your life. It is a record of self-discovery.

Though this workbook is designed to be written in, sometimes you may need or want more space. Please dedicate a separate journal or notebook to write or draw more extensively about your experiences with daily practices and mindful art encounters. Some of the encounters suggest the use of additional materials, such as collaging materials or brush-and-ink. These are valuable experiences, but please feel at liberty to adapt these to the materials you have on hand.

Each chapter of the workbook starts with some reflections about and intentions for the week's work. Think of these pages as setting the table for the practice, exercises, and opportunities for exploration that follow.

This is followed by the week's Daily Practice outline, a list of the daily practices, exercises, and experiments that I recommend each week. These include art exercises, journaling, meditation, yoga, and movement practices. You can use this to plan your routine for each week: when you will do your body-centered practices, which art experiences you'll do on which days, what materials you may want or need. If there is anything you'll need to print out or download for the chapter, I'll mention it here.

Then come the Mindful Art Encounters. Most of the chapters teach between three and six of these, for a total of thirty-five suggested encounters. Since you'll do one per day while you are working your way through the nine-week program, sometimes you will do an experience more than once. You'll likely notice that the experience changes each time you do it.

Each chapter rounds out with an invitation for you to reflect upon your week's journey before moving on to the next chapter.

As you work through the program, feel free to adjust your routines according to whatever you feel is most helpful and useful. For example, trying the same exercise at different times of day (or night) can give you new experiences and insights. Strapped for time? Take your workbook and journal in your bag and weave it into your busy life. And even though this is designed as a nine-week program, you can also do the Mindful Art Encounters out of sequence if you feel inspired to do so, or repeat them as many times as you choose, or even add your own variations and explorations (see "A Few Final Notes," below).

The first encounters are designed to be done on your own without outside distraction so you can listen to your inner dialogue. Later, after you have experienced the encounters alone, additional encounters are added to be shared with a partner and others with a group.

May this book bring hours of playful exploration and learning, curiosity, surprise, wise understanding, fun, joy, and meaningfulness. May each moment lead to the spilling over of presence and acceptance of life exactly as it is, welcoming change as it unfolds from moment to moment. You may discover that this journey is an artistic expression of life living through you as you celebrate the profound gift that is *now*.

A FEW FINAL NOTES

The exercises in this workbook are intended to be repeated, allowing for learning through practice and deep play, rather than as entertaining, one-time experiences. Most of these encounters take about ten to fifteen minutes to complete—take longer if you like.

With practice, you'll deepen your connection to the process, discovering an inner rhythm that is genuine and personal and feels like it is flowing rather than imposing. You may grow and broaden your horizon, building resilience and confidence in your ability to express yourself uniquely.

As you work through each week's practice, keep the following suggested guidelines in mind:

- Commit six days each week to your mindful appointments with yourself (even if only for five minutes). If you have difficulty keeping your appointments, write a note to yourself.

- When feeling rushed or distracted, bring your attention back to the breath, remembering the acronym STOP: Stop; Take a breath; Observe what is felt and sensed; Proceed with awareness.

- When engaging in the practices, turn off your cell phone and make sure that you will not be disturbed. Wear comfortable clothing and remove your shoes.

- Trust the process.

And remember: rather than not practice at all, create a practice that works for you at this time. Be creative in your choice and stretch your ability and comfort. Rather than falling into habitual patterns of practice, find the place where intention, fresh learning, insight, and discipline all come together. Venture into new ways that may turn you inside out and stretch you into new realms. For example, rather than retreating from and resisting a moment of discomfort, you may find that you become curious about your options. Always listen to what feels right and, rather than adhere to instructions, let your inner voice of self compassion guide you in a healthy and generous way.

Allow yourself to embrace and enjoy the gift of self-expression. Life is precious and there's no time to waste, so leave your mark.

Who Am I?

The mind in its natural state can be compared to the sky, covered by layers of cloud which hide its true nature.

—Kalu Rinpoche, *Real Life Mindfulness* by Becca Anderson

The journey of self-discovery begins wherever you are. The first step is bringing awareness to the breath happening moment to moment. This process—breathing—begins when we are born and continues until we die. It requires nothing from us. It is automatic and connects us to the present moment and the experience of being alive. Breathing in and out—we experience this process through the body. The breath enters and is received by the body and then leaves as the body releases it and lets it go. There is no technique to learn.

Begin by taking a few deep breaths. Feel the breath, the body, and the breath in the body. Investigate the interconnected process of receiving and releasing your breath and the rhythm of the process. Feel the temperature of the air as it enters your nostrils. (Is it warm or cool?) Feel the texture of the breath as it flows in on the inhalation, following the process to the end of the inhalation. Perhaps noticing the pause at the end of the inhalation, before beginning the exhalation. Bring awareness to your breath starting *now*. The past has already gone. The future has not yet arrived. Discovery is in the present.

No matter what circumstances or challenges you are facing, there is more right with you than wrong with you. You are more than enough, and you have all the resources within to begin your journey of discovery. This week is about awakening to your innate wholeness and the notion that you are "enough"—more than enough! It is about deepening your understanding of who you are in this moment. You will begin to explore the question, "Who am I?" through art and body-centered practices. The fact is, you are perfect just the way you are. You are whole and an exquisite being no matter how broken you feel.

Self-discovery is a journey in understanding your life more fully and deeply, inviting meaning, acceptance, and kindness. It is the freedom to choose your perspective and respond, rather than react, to your circumstances. It is a chance to affirm who you are and to live a genuine, authentic, engaged life. It is the opportunity to move through the unscripted moments of life, engaged, alive, alert, aware, and awake; to be unrehearsed, fresh, and new.

As you begin to discover "the self," you are also on a journey to discover and understand that you are not alone. You are connected to others in this human experience. We all share our humanity and the experience of being alive. And as you relate to yourself in a more loving, kind, and compassionate way, this inner knowing can spill and ripple out into the rest of your life—into relationships, community, and connection to nature, animals, and the interconnected world. The inner work you do is not selfish—it benefits us all.

This work is the most important in this lifetime. Who are you? How can understanding who you are change your life? And in a larger context, how can understanding who you are change the world? What do you want to do with this one precious life?

The first step is to ask the question: Who am I in this moment? Shine a light on understanding who you are *now*. You are not trying to change anything. You are only bringing kind understanding to your inner knowing. And as you befriend the experiences of sadness, loss, anger, jealousy, love, fear, illness, and suffering, you are able to empathize with others. These experiences are our common threads, weaving color and texture through our lives as we respond accordingly.

In our lives, we often try to achieve a state of "getting it right." But life is not about getting it right. Life is an opportunity for understanding our true nature. We invite all experiences as opportunities to practice letting go of attachment, to wake up and experience life moment to moment. In this way, we give ourselves the possibility of greater freedom and choice. By practicing awareness of where your attention is, you can deliberately choose to respond creatively rather than react out of habitual patterns.

Let's begin this process, this creative journey of exploring new ways of being and relating. First is an exercise in inventorying and naming feelings.

Mindfulness is developed by purposefully paying attention in a sustained and nonjudgmental way to what is going on in your body, your mind, and in the world around you. It is about being awake and aware, living in the present, simply being yourself and knowing something about who that is.

—Jon Kabat-Zinn, *Full Catastrophe Living*

FEELINGS INVENTORY: TUNING IN TO THE LANGUAGE OF THE BODY

As we move through this journey of self-discovery, we will be investigating and becoming familiar with emotional states, physical sensations, and thoughts, experienced moment to moment. It may be helpful to familiarize yourself with terms to describe what you're feeling.

The following are words we use when we want to express a combination of *emotional states* and *physical sensations*, engaging a process of deepening self-discovery and facilitating greater understanding and connection to self and others.

There are two parts to this list: feelings you may have when your needs are being met and feelings you may have when your needs are *not* being met. What words have resonance for you right now, as you enter this journey? Circle the words that feel true. With each lesson, refer back to these lists to help identify your specific emotions and body sensations. In this process, you will begin to learn the difference between your emotions and sensations in your body.

Feelings When Your Needs Are Satisfied

AFFECTIONATE	ENGAGED	EXCITED	PEACEFUL
compassionate	alert	amazed	calm
friendly	curious	eager	centered
loving	fascinated	energetic	comfortable
open-hearted	interested	enthusiastic	content
sympathetic	intrigued	lively	equanimous
tender	involved	passionate	fulfilled
warm	stimulated	vibrant	quiet
			trusting
CONFIDENT	**EXHILARATED**	**HOPEFUL**	
empowered	appreciative	encouraged	**REFRESHED**
open	blissful	expectant	enlivened
proud	elated	optimistic	rejuvenated
safe	exuberant		renewed
secure	moved	**JOYFUL**	rested
	radiant	amused	restored
INSPIRED	thankful	delighted	revived
amazed	thrilled	glad	
awed		happy	
wonder-filled		jubilant	
		pleased	

Feelings When Your Needs Are Not Satisfied

AFRAID

dreading

frightened

mistrustful

panicked

scared

suspicious

terrified

worried

ANNOYED

aggravated

disgruntled

displeased

exasperated

frustrated

impatient

irritated

ANGRY

enraged

furious

incensed

indignant

judged

judgmental

outraged

resentful

EMBARRASSED

ashamed

flustered

guilty

mortified

self-conscious

CONFUSED

ambivalent

baffled

bewildered

dazed

hesitant

lost

perplexed

DISCONNECTED

alienated

bored

cold

detached

distant

distracted

indifferent

numb

uninterested

withdrawn

DISQUIETED

agitated

disturbed

restless

shocked

startled

surprised

in turmoil

uncomfortable

uneasy

unsettled

upset

FATIGUED

burnt out

depleted

exhausted

lethargic

listless

sleepy

tired

worn out

IN PAIN

devastated

grief-stricken

heartbroken

hurt

lonely

miserable

regretful

remorseful

REPELLED

contemptuous

disdainful

disgusted

hateful

horrified

hostile

repulsed

unfriendly

YEARNING

envious

jealous

SAD

depressed

in despair

disappointed

discouraged

disheartened

heavy hearted

hopeless

unhappy

TENSE

anxious

cranky

fidgety

frazzled

irritable

nervous

overwhelmed

restless

stressed out

VULNERABLE

fragile

guarded

helpless

insecure

leery

reserved

sensitive

shaky

List of Needs

AUTONOMY

choice

freedom

independence

space

spontaneity

CONNECTION

acceptance

affection

appreciation

closeness

communication

community

companionship

compassion

cooperation

empathy

love

nurturing

respect/self-respect

safety

security

stability

support

trust

understanding

warmth

witnessing

HONESTY

authenticity

integrity

presence

MEANING

awareness

belonging

celebrating life

challenge

clarity

competence

consciousness

contribute

creativity

discovery

growth

hope

learning

mourning

purpose

self-expression

understanding

PEACE

beauty

communion

ease

equality

harmony

inspiration

order

PHYSICAL WELL-BEING

air

exercise

food

rest/sleep

safety/shelter

sensual expression

touch

water

PLAY

joy

humor

Feelings Inventory © 2005 by Center for Nonviolent Communication, http://www.cnvc.org (email: cnvc@cnvc.org; tel: 505-244-4041)

WEEK 1 INTENTIONS

During this first week of the MBSE program, you will commit:

- To meet yourself as if for the very first time, learning who you innately are rather than who you think you *should* be.

- To become familiar with the breath and a daily mindfulness practice.

- To work with your body to start examining and exploring your direct experience of feelings, emotions, and the senses.

- To become aware of your thoughts, both positive and negative.

WEEK 1 DAILY PRACTICE

The list below details your practice for week 1. Read through the list and, if you like, use it to prepare in advance for the week's practice—for instance, by deciding on and noting which Mindful Art Encounters you'd like to do on which days, and so on. You can download a printable version of this list at http://www. newharbinger.com/44932 and post it in a place where you can see it easily. Visit the same URL to download the Art of Mindfulness Practice Guide, which contains directions for the body scan and gentle stretching yoga. (Audio guides for these practices are available there, too.)

1. Do one of the Mindful Art Encounters that follow every day. Some you will do more than once.

2. Practice the body scan at least six times this week. See the downloadable Art of Mindfulness Practice Guide for body scan instructions.

3. A few times a day, pause in your activities and bring full awareness to the present moment. Note sounds arising, whatever thoughts there may be, emotions, and what you are seeing in your surroundings. Bring your attention to sensations in your body and the experience of your breath. Allow yourself to become present to what is actually happening for several moments. Rest in the space effortlessly, pausing and then returning to the task at hand. Notice the effect this has as you proceed. When you have a moment to do so, record your thoughts in your journal, or in the Record of Mindful Moments log found in the downloadable Art of Mindfulness Practice Guide.

4. Take a few minutes each day to do some gentle stretching yoga. Depending on your schedule, you can just do a few stretches, or you can use the gentle yoga practice guide found in the downloadable Art of Mindfulness Practice Guide.

5. Work with the nine dots puzzle (in the next section).

6. This week, try to eat a meal, a snack, or even just a few bites with mindful attention on the experience. (You will learn a formal mindful eating practice next week.)

7. Consider the question, "Who am I?" throughout the week before engaging in the body scan, when transitioning from one activity to another, and whenever you remember. Notice what arises in the space of asking the question.

8. Make a daily gratitude list. Each morning, write down five things you are grateful for as you begin the day. Then, in the evening as you recall your day, list five more things.

9. At the end of the week, complete the Reflecting on the Week section at the end of this chapter.

Nine Dots

Try to connect the nine dots below using four straight lines, without lifting your pencil or pen off the page or retracing any of the lines. After working on the puzzle for a while—whether or not you have solved it—read the explanation that follows.

Explanation: The nine dots exercise is a useful way to explore how we typically solve problems in a habitual way. For example, our efforts might follow one or more of the following patterns:

1. We try over and over to solve the problem and do not give up, but always stay in the same groove. We repeat similar efforts over and over.

2. We give up easily and go to the Internet to find the solution.

3. We experiment with creating a new way of solving the puzzle. By expanding perception and thinking out of the box, we may break free from self-imposed limitations, creating new understanding.

This is an opportunity to see whether you tend to spend a great deal of effort trying to solve problems using well-trodden, habitual patterns. Or do you give up easily and seek outside help? Or do you employ creative ways of risking, exploring, and trying new solutions?

Similarly, this exercise sheds light on whether we are stuck in habits and a notion of who we are. By asking the question, "Who am I?" we have an opportunity to see that who we are is changing moment-to-moment and how we choose to solve problems can be a creative encounter inspired by the present moment, filled with possibility, surprise, and new out-of-the-box perceptions. (This puzzle has several possible solutions: to see them, type "nine-dots solution" into a search engine.)

Mindful Art Encounter #1: Who Am I?

Materials: Pencil or pen; journal

List twenty words answering the question: Who am I? With curiosity and friendliness, list the words that come to you immediately, as if you were describing yourself to a stranger. This is our chance to look at who we are in this moment in time, as we begin our MBSE journey.

We'll revisit this exercise again at the end, in week 9, to see how our knowing of who we are may have changed.

1. _____

2. _____

3. _____

4. _____

5. _____

6. _____

7. _____

8. _____

9. _____

10. _____

11. _____

12. _____

13. _____

14. _____

15. _____

16. _____

17. _____

18. _____

19. _____

20. _____

Now write your responses to the questions below. If you need more space to write, use your journal.

How creative are you?

_____

_____

_____

_____

What is your relationship to creativity and the creative process?

_____

_____

_____

_____

What role does creativity play in your everyday life?

_____

_____

_____

_____

Mindful Art Encounter #2: Finding Your Personal Mark

Materials: Paper and pencil, journal

We all have the ability to make simple marks or strokes with a pencil, but amazingly, we all make them differently. Our marks are acts of personal expression, like our handwriting. In this exercise, the seemingly simple process of mark-making may help you break through the ice of creativity. For the sake of paring down the process, the suggestion is to use just a pencil.

There is no right way or wrong way to express your authentic mark. We're simply exercising familiarity with our mark, making it repetitively on the page as we breathe in and out.

Beginning in one corner at the top of a blank page, make a short vertical line. Repeat the mark over and over in a row across the page, until you reach the opposite corner. All of the lines should be similar length, similar direction, and similar distance apart on the page.

As you may soon notice, little imagination or creativity is required to do this. The practice is repetition. When you finish the row, drop down and make a second row of the same marks. Repeat for ten to fifteen rows. When the page is filled and you have made the final mark, pause.

When you finish, put the pencil down and take three deep breaths. Close your eyes and feel what is to be felt in the body. Bring awareness to the present moment. Experience it all without judgment, allowing it to be just as it is, without trying to change it. Now write your responses to the questions below. If you need more space to write, use your journal.

What did you notice in the experience of repetition in the mark-making process?

_____

_____

_____

What did you sense or feel in your body?

_____

_____

What emotions arose in the process?

_____

_____

What did you learn?

_____

_____

_____

Did you sense a connection between your mark-making and the inhalation and exhalation of your breath?

_____

_____

Observe the fifteen rows of lines. As you look closely, consider the following::

- What did you discover as you practiced repetition?

_____

_____

- Did anything change along the way?

_____

_____

- What do you notice about your marks?

_____

_____

In the simple moments, there are gifts we can learn. We do not need to have big things happen to appreciate our lives. We can find enjoyment within simple moments, such as the making of lines. Repetition can be healing. Allow playful experimentation, even in what might seem like a "simple" repetitive exercise, and ask yourself: What can I learn? How might I be surprised?

If you would like to do this exercise again, feel free to re-create it on a blank page. Any time you repeat this exercise, journal about your experience.

Mindful Art Encounter #3: Exploring Your Personal Mark

Materials: Paper and pencil, journal

You may have now become more familiar with your mark-making process. You are about to expand the inquiry, introducing the element of variation. Now let's explore the process of repetition and variation, engaging imagination, creativity, innovation, and play.

Beginning in one corner at the top of a blank page, make a mark. This time, keep all the marks similar in length but introduce variation in direction. Make some of your marks vertical, others horizontal or diagonal. Vary the distance between each mark. Vary as many things as you can imagine, repeating the mark over and over in a row across the page until you reach the opposite corner. You're now engaging imagination, creativity, innovation, and play with repetition and variation.

When you finish the first row, drop down and make a second row, introducing different directions and relationships, rhythms, groupings, spacing, hard versus soft marks and thick versus thin. Repeat for fifteen rows.

As you play with possibility of repetition and variation, let the process unfold without goals and preconceived ideas. Stay present with each mark in each moment, engaging a quality of aliveness. Let go of it needing to be a certain way. Let go of perfection. Let the process reveal itself in each moment. Play and have fun.

How do repetition, variation, and rhythm feel? You might find that a particular rhythm or pattern emerges, perhaps even one related to the rhythm of your breath, the rhythm of your heart beating, or the rhythm of you walking in the world.

As you experiment with the repetitive process, adding variation, notice your inner dialogue.

There is no right or wrong way to express your authentic mark. You're simply exercising familiarity with the process of mark-making, repetition, and variation. When your mind wanders, just notice that it has wandered off and then, without judgment, gently and firmly bring it back to the present moment of mark-making.

When you finish, put the pencil down and take three deep breaths. Close your eyes and notice what you feel in your body. Once again, inquire into this moment of having completed the exercise. Notice your inner dialogue.

Respond to the questions below; if you need more space to write, use your journal.

- Did you feel a sense of play? _____

- Were you surprised in any way? _____

Observe the fifteen rows of lines. Respond to the questions below; if you need more space to write, use your journal.

- Is each mark unique? _____

- Engage slowly, looking and noticing. What do you see?

  _____

  _____

  _____

- Is there a particular pattern that emerged naturally?

  _____

  _____

As you introduced variation in direction and grouping, how did this change the process? Were you engaged in imagination at play, or thinking about needing to "get it right"?

_____

_____

_____

What did you notice as you began to explore variation? Were you aware of thinking?

_____

_____

_____

_____

Through this second mark-making encounter, you may begin to recognize your inner dialogue: maybe how much you judge yourself, how critical you are, or how you feel uncomfortable experimenting without being focused on outcome. Many of us are used to following instructions and outer directives, and working without them can bring up fear and discomfort. Experience it all without judgment, allowing it to be just as it is, without trying to change it.

Any time you repeat this exercise, journal about your experience.

Mindful Art Encounter #4: Freedom of Self-Expression

Materials: Paper and pencil, journal

This time let's invite even more imagination, creativity, and freedom into your mark-making, spontaneously and without any guidelines.

Begin by making a mark—any mark—anywhere on a blank page, and then continue mark-making in a free and playful way. Each mark inspires the next. Staying aware of your breath, play with curiosity. Use lines of any length and width, straight or curvy, rounded shapes or squares and rectangles, irregular shapes, dots of any size and distance apart, shapes of any size and form. Position your marks anywhere on the page and introduce any other means and variation of marks that come out of spontaneity. There is no right way or wrong way to express your authentic mark.

Begin to create a visual expression, letting a conversation emerge, mark by mark, on the page. There is no plan, no goal, no preconceived idea. You are simply communicating to yourself who you are in this moment through marks. Stay open to risk and surprise, following the thread one mark at a time. As you engage playfully, imaginatively, and creatively, surprise and wonder may arise. This process invites presence in each moment, engaging a quality of aliveness. Let go of all past experience and stand in the process. As you continue, what are you noticing? What is changing? Are you relating and befriending—or resisting?

When your mind wanders, notice what types of thoughts come into your mind, and then gently return to your mark-making.

When you finish, put the pencil down and take three deep breaths. Close your eyes and notice what you feel in the body. Take a few more deep breaths.

Now respond to the questions below; if you need more space to write, use your journal.

- What has changed? How was your experience similar or different this time?

_____

_____

_____

_____

- Were you aware of thinking?

  _____

- Did you experience moments of playful engagement? How did this feel?

  _____

  _____

  _____

  _____

  _____

  _____

- Did you notice a judging mind or an evaluating mind?

  _____

Any time you repeat this exercise, respond to the questions in your journal.

Mindful Art Encounter #5: Body Scan Self-Portrait

Materials: Colored pencils, pens, or crayons; journal

Note: Before starting this exercise, review the guide for the body scan meditation in the downloadable Art of Mindfulness Practice Guide found at http://www.newharbinger.com/44932.

One of the most important tools in our journey is the body scan, designed to bring greater awareness of the body just as it is in the present moment. We allow ourselves to fully experience our body's moment-to-moment conditions through noticing and listening, without judgment, words or story. Using all of our senses—hearing, tasting, seeing, touching, and smelling—we experience the richness of the world in our own uniquely attuned senses. This is an exercise we'll return to repeatedly throughout the book.

Start by doing a body scan, following the downloadable print or audio guide. You may feel certain things in your body, such as constriction, freedom, stiffness, or pain. Befriend and allow all of these sensations.

When you've finished the scan, use colored pencils or crayons to fill in the body outline on the next page, expressing your experience directly rather than thinking about it. What physical sensations, thoughts, and/or emotions arose most prominently for you? Use color, line, shape, and form. Avoid words or recognizable symbols or representations, allowing the expression to be abstract.

There is no right or wrong in this exercise. This type of drawing has been with humanity from time immemorial, going back thousands of years to cave paintings. The process of drawing and mark-making is a primordial form of human communication. Give yourself the opportunity to explore and be curious.

The practice is to be with all experience without editing or needing to change it in any way, being aware of all experience even if your mind is wandering over and over again. Wandering thoughts, emotions, and sensations are all part of the process. Notice the passing events. If a critical or judging voice arises, simply notice it and return to the vibrancy of the present moment of drawing, colors, lines, and shapes. If you have trouble remembering what you felt, close your eyes and reconnect with part of the body scan. Then, when you're ready, continue the drawing.

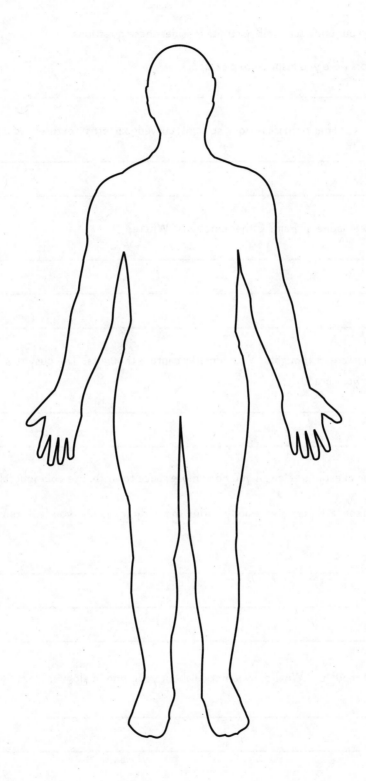

After drawing your body scan self-portrait, consider these questions:

- What colors were you inspired to pick up?

  _____

- What types of lines or marks—dots, straight, curved, patterns, textures— did you make?

  _____

  _____

- Did you feel sadness? Pain? Other emotions? Where?

  _____

  _____

  _____

- Were you aware of thoughts? Which marks capture thoughts? The busyness in your head? The rhythm of your breath?

  _____

  _____

Respond to the questions below; if you need more space to write, use your journal.

Were you able to feel each part of the body during the body scan? Did you feel some areas more than others?

_____

_____

_____

Were you aware of thoughts? What did you notice about your inner dialogue?

_____

_____

_____

Were you distracted from physical sensations by thoughts? Emotions? Were you aware of sleepiness or the mind wandering?

_____

_____

Were you aware of similar past experiences as you engaged with drawing?

_____

_____

Were you able to feel your breath in your body? Where did you feel the breath most vividly?

_____

Did you feel pain, tension, or discomfort? Where?

_____

_____

Was it helpful to express your feelings, emotions, and thoughts visually?

_____

What did you learn during the body scan and portrait? Were you surprised by anything?

_____

_____

_____

_____

Any time you repeat this exercise, you can download and print out a blank body scan portrait sheet at http://www.newharbinger.com/44932, and respond to the reflection questions in your journal.

REFLECTING ON THE WEEK

When you finish the week's work, take some time to reflect before going on. Write in your journal or on the blank lines on whichever of the reflections or prompts below speak to you.

Reflections

- Through practice we learn to connect with direct experience.

- You are an exquisite being, and as long as you're breathing, there is far more right than wrong with you, whatever you may think is wrong with you.

- By connecting with your breath, body sensations, and emotions, you may begin to investigate and connect with life experience more deeply.

Journal Prompts

What are your own reflections of this week? What have you learned? In particular, what have you learned about your inner dialogue, your relationships with others, and your relationship to self-compassion, experimentation, patience, and curiosity?

_____

_____

_____

_____

_____

_____

_____

_____

_____

_____

How will this experience inform your life going forward? What would you like to incorporate into your daily practice? What would you like to let go of?

_____

_____

_____

_____

_____

_____

_____

_____

What did you learn about your experience this week that you particularly want to remember?

_____

_____

_____

_____

_____

_____

_____

After you have written, close your eyes and notice the sensations in your body, emotions, and thoughts.

Week 2

Opening to Your Reality

Meditation is the only intentional systematic human activity which at bottom is about not trying to improve yourself or get anywhere else, but simply to realize where you already are.

—Jon Kabat-Zinn, *Wherever You Go, There You Are*

Perception shapes our lives. We see things through the lens of our personal perspective, and this then determines how we respond to everything. Perception is rooted in experience beginning in childhood. Our reality is learned through values reflected in our family, community, and the world around us, resulting in a learned and habitual dance of liking versus not liking, pleasant versus unpleasant, responding versus resisting. We begin to build a construct of our lives. If we accept this construct, it can keep us stuck in a familiar box of habits, judgments, prejudice, and expectations arising from our learned perception of relatedness with ourselves, others, society, nature, and the world we live in.

How often do you operate out of expectations? When we're in the comfort zone of habit, rehashing and rehearsing (or "re-" anything) what is expected and familiar, nothing really happens to expand our perceptions. We may go around and around in the same patterns. Many of us constantly assess, compare, and evaluate based on our "fixed" perceptions, finding things not quite right, not good enough, compared to what we want them to be. These perceptions and expectations can keep us suffering rather than opening our perception to accept things as they are.

But, in fact, your power of perception can expand into a wider view. Your mind can accept, rather than try to change, what you perceive to be unpleasant, recognizing that you can have pleasant moments in spite of being in crisis and pain and unpleasant moments in situations that would normally be perceived as pleasurable.

Mindfulness is about loosening the need for control and for things to be a certain way; instead it is spaciously receiving *all* experience—even challenging moments and times of loss—as an integral part of life. This is an important way of learning about our attitude and our willingness to start again. Perception

Maybe, Said the Farmer

Zen parable, author unknown

Once upon a time there was an old farmer who had worked his crops for many years. One day, his horse ran away. Upon hearing the news, his neighbors came to visit. "Such bad luck," they said sympathetically.

"Maybe," the farmer replied.

The next morning the horse returned, bringing with it three other wild horses. "How wonderful," the neighbors exclaimed.

"Maybe," replied the old man.

The following day, his son tried to ride one of the untamed horses, was thrown, and broke his leg. The neighbors again came to offer their sympathy on his misfortune.

"Maybe," answered the farmer.

The day after, military officials came to the village to draft young men into the army. Seeing that the son's leg was broken, they passed him by. The neighbors congratulated the farmer on how well things had turned out.

"Maybe," said the farmer.

is limitless, spacious, personal, and highly experiential. If we open to see more spaciously with alert awareness—approaching life with humility and a beginner's mind—we can let go of rigid judgments and fixed views of what is good or bad, pleasant or unpleasant. A beginner's mind is similar to the mind of a child. Each moment is an opportunity to begin again and see things with the neutral eyes of a child rather than seeing habitually through the perspective learned over time. It is a state of playful engagement, driven by firsthand experience through our senses and our body, rather than *thinking* about the experience.

Once we do this, we may begin to understand perception more fully, seeing it as a breathing, moving process that changes as we open our view. We may learn to recognize our reactivity and see that we have choices about how to respond, especially when things in our lives fall apart.

When your life takes an unexpected turn—for example, through the end of a relationship, loss of a job, death of a loved one, health issues, or moving—mindfulness offers you a way to strengthen your inner resources and affirm that you can, in fact, begin again. This does not mean you will not feel loss and sadness, but that you will have practiced your coping skills and will be able to better *choose* how to respond, rather than simply react in old, unhelpful ways. Rather than being a victim of circumstance, you can respond mindfully, riding the waves of uncertainty and loss with greater ease and well-being. Mindfulness invites you to shed your old outer layers and enter a new space of self compassion, accepting things as they are, engaging with core strength and inner wisdom.

You can assume responsibility in your life by:

- learning to self-reflect with kindness

- listening to the language of your body: thoughts, emotions, and body sensations

- choosing health-enhancing behaviors and overall well-being

- recognizing self-defeating habits

- building informal mindfulness practices into your daily routine to engage with life in the present.

- building your creative "muscles" so you may experience life as a constantly unfolding creative expression.

Being in life is, in fact, a constantly unfolding act of creative expression. Think of it as painting a canvas of your life and living it stroke by stroke, mark by mark. It is a personal journey that is unique to each of us. Each moment, you have the opportunity to paint a stroke of reactivity, fighting and resisting, or to choose to create music, singing and dancing with the joy of being fully alive, awake, and open. Just as we do cardio and endurance training to prepare for a marathon, practicing mindfulness is training for the marathon of life, building our creative muscles and aligning our core rhythm, intuition, values, intention, and vision as we embrace our truth from within. When you are strong, you are like a mountain: present, rooted, and firmly grounded in all weather. The mountain retains its "mountain-ness" through storms, tsunamis, blizzards, floods, sunshine, and darkness.

This week, we'll explore the foundational concept of perception as the root of all experience. Through art encounters and mindfulness practices, we will identify expectations, judgments, prejudice, and rules that keep us on automatic pilot, stuck in a fixed reality that may not serve us anymore.

In addition to the body scan, which you'll continue doing daily, this week you'll introduce brief periods of sitting meditation as a way to integrate mindfulness into daily living. Meditation involves working with the "wandering mind," a universal phenomenon of all human brains. Working with and accepting the wandering mind is an essential part of mindfulness practice. The refocusing of attention and "coming back" are as much part of meditation as is staying on the object of attention. By paying attention to what is on your mind and where your mind goes, you will become better able to accept your thoughts and feelings, reducing the tendency to *force* things to be a certain way. This exercise in "letting be" is a new way of engaging in the world.

Perception is the material with which we paint our reality. If you choose the colors and textures with imagination, courage, self compassion, and a willingness to be open, you can create a masterpiece. Stand in your color and sing your life!

WEEK 2 INTENTIONS

During this week of the MBSE program, you will be:

- Observing how perception shapes your views and can keep you stuck on automatic pilot, even when it no longer serves you.

- Challenging your need for control and start opening up to all experience, the pleasant or unpleasant, and the neutral or in between.

- To start seeing how even loss and sadness can lead to possibility and growth.

WEEK 2 DAILY PRACTICE

The list below details your practice for week 2. Read through it and, if you like, use it to prepare in advance for the week's practice—for instance, by deciding on and noting which Mindful Art Encounters you'd like to do on which days, reviewing new meditations (such as this week's sitting meditation), and gathering materials. You can download a printable version of this list at http://www.newharbinger. com/44932 and post it in a place where you can see it easily. Visit the same URL to download the Art of Mindfulness Practice Guide, which contains printable files of the directions for the body scan, sitting meditation, and gentle stretching yoga. (Audio guides for these practices are available there, too, as are printable PDFs of the Pleasant and Unpleasant Events Calendars and the Record of Mindful Moments.)

1. Do the week 2 Mindful Art Encounters (in the sections that follow) in order, starting with Encounter #6 and ending with Encounter #9. Do no more than one Encounter in a single day.

2. Do the formal mindful eating practice found in this chapter.

3. Practice the body scan each day. Do this exercise without expectations; allow yourself to feel what you feel without attempting to judge or change it. Write about your experiences in your journal.

4. Do a sitting meditation for ten minutes per day. See the downloadable Art of Mindfulness Practice Guide for instructions.

5. Add one entry each day to the Pleasant Events and Unpleasant Events calendars. (Copy these from the back of the book or download the PDFs.)

6. Continue to bring mindfulness to routine activities, such as brushing your teeth, checking the mail, washing dishes, taking a shower, taking out the garbage, shopping, and eating. Pause in the activity and bring full awareness to the present moment. Note sounds, thoughts, emotions, and what you are seeing. Bring your attention to sensations in your body. Rest in the space, and then return to the activity. Notice the effect this has as you proceed. Later, write your thoughts in the Record of Mindful Moments. (Copy this from the back of the book or download the PDF.)

7. Continue writing a daily gratitude list in your journal. Each morning, write down five things you are grateful for as you begin the day. Then, in the evening as you recall your day, list five more things.

8. Complete the Reflecting on the Week section at the end of this chapter.

Tips for Turning Your Attention Inward

Mindfulness involves turning your attention inward. Here are some ways to focus on your inner dialogue in everyday life:

1. Do a ten-minute sitting meditation, simply focusing on your breath.

2. Open spaces in your life for silence and non-doing.

3. Practice bringing your attention to the present moment: breathing in and breathing out periodically throughout the day.

4. Eat a meal in silence.

5. Bring awareness to sounds in the moment. Listen, engage, and be with the sounds.

6. Decide not to turn on the television or radio.

7. Engage with art—whether a Mindful Art Encounter or any creative activity, such as cooking, gardening, arranging flowers—as a doorway to understanding life more fully.

8. Become aware of distractions and how they take you away from your inner dialogue, alienating you from experiencing your life in the present moment. Choose how you allow distractions into your life and learn how to say no. (For more on this, see the "No" Practice in week 3.)

9. Sprinkle seeds of self compassion, kindness and generosity over all experience.

10. Take care of yourself.

Mindful Eating

What you will need: A single raisin or other bite-sized food

When you eat a meal, do you experience it with all of your senses? Or do you eat while distracted—watching TV, using your phone, or just thinking about the future or past? Do you eat quickly, or do you savor each bite, chewing slowly? Do you eat to quiet an emotion or soothe a worry or anxiety?

Eating is a practice we do each day, offering a frequent opportunity for practicing informal mindfulness. In this exercise, we'll learn how to bring mindfulness to any meal—in this case, mindfully eating a raisin.

Place a raisin (or any edible object) in the palm of your hand. Imagine that you are from another planet. You have just landed on Earth, and you have never seen such an object before. You are curious and begin to explore the object with all of your senses.

Seeing:

- Focus your attention, and with curiosity—as if you have never seen this object before—really looking at it.

- Pay attention to its color.

- Notice areas that are catching the light.

- Look at it carefully and investigate areas of light and dark, reflections and shadows, ridges and grooves.

Touching:

- Take the object between two fingers.

- Explore the textures, noticing if it is smooth or rough, soft or hard.

- Turn the object around, noticing variations on each side.

Smelling:

- Bring the object closer to your nose, noticing the smell.

Hearing:

- Bring the object to one ear and roll it between your fingers, noticing if there is any sound.

Tasting:

- Slowly bring the object to your mouth, noticing what happens inside your mouth. Is saliva forming? Gently place the object in your mouth, resting it on the tongue without biting. What is the sensation of the object in your mouth?

- When you're ready, bite down on the object, noticing how the teeth get into position for a bite to take place. After the bite, what is the sensation of taste? Slowly begin to chew the object, bringing your awareness to the process. What are you noticing? Being aware of saliva mixing with the object and notice how the consistency and taste change as you chew. When you are ready to swallow, note the intention to swallow and then bring awareness to swallowing. Is it possible to follow the changing sensations of swallowing the object and it traveling down your throat into the esophagus and into your stomach? Pause and take a moment to congratulate yourself for taking the time to experience mindful eating.

When thoughts arise, notice that you are thinking (*Ah! I'm thinking.*) and then gently and firmly bring your attention back to the object. This noticing is a mindful moment. You are training the mind to come back again and again to the present moment and to invite all experience firsthand, rather than through thought and intellect.

Now reflect on your experience, and answer the questions below, using your journal if you need more space to write.

- What are you aware of learning?

- Were you surprised in any way?

- Did you notice any habit that you were not aware of?

- What did you notice about your relationship to food and eating?

- Do you enjoy eating?

- In trying to see this object as if for the very first time without any preconceptions, what did you learn?

_____

_____

_____

_____

_____

_____

_____

_____

_____

Moving forward, as you approach each meal, try:

- pausing before taking your first bite to observe the food

- appreciating where the food has come from: all the different processes that had to occur to bring this food to your plate, from the seed that was planted to the weather, soil, farmers' market, factories, packaging, stores, and then your effort to purchase it

- feeling a sense of appreciation for all the effort and energy required to present you with food and how nature and humans are interconnected and interdependent.

Mindful Art Encounter #6: Conversation Drawing with Self

Materials: Paper and any art materials that speak to your creative process, such as pencil, glue, paint, crayons, pastels, or even non-art materials such as sticks, flowers, sand, leaves, recycled objects, and so on; pen or pencil; journal

Building on the exercises from week 1, this "conversation drawing" with yourself encourages a broader range of exploring and experimenting, inviting courage, risk-taking, imagining, creating, and, most importantly, *playing.* There is great learning in repetition, which is why we call it "practice" and not "perfection." In repetition, we deepen our inquiry and may become familiar with our hidden habits as well as things that bring us joy and a sense of connection to our core.

This exercise is done in silence. Make sure all technology is turned off and that you will not be disturbed. Remember, this is an appointment with yourself. Just as you make time for appointments with others, honor this time alone. Notice how you respond to (or resist) the alone time.

If relevant, let your family, partner, or friend know that you will be out of reach for twenty minutes so they are aware of and respect your space. If done regularly, this boundary-setting will spill over into other areas of your life, too. Taking time for yourself and approaching the process of discovering and understanding your life more deeply with kind attention, curiosity, and commitment is essential to create a happy life.

Begin by closing your eyes or lowering your gaze. Take three deep breaths. Feel the sensations and rhythm of inhalation and exhalation in your body. With curiosity and practice, you may find that you begin to build an intimate relationship with your process of breathing.

- Where are you feeling the process of breathing most vividly?

- Is it in your nostrils, feeling the air as it enters on the inhalation and as it leaves on the exhalation?

- Or is it your chest, rising and expanding on the inhalation and falling on the exhalation?

- Or are you feeling it more deeply in the belly, expanding like a balloon on the inhalation and deflating on the exhalation?

Feel into the body, receive, and release the air in an automatic, natural rhythm that needs no effort. Notice if your mind wanders away from the breath. Pause and then come back to the breath in the body.

Before beginning your conversation drawing, affirm your intention to be present and listen deeply to the experience of life in all its colors and dimensions through the language of experience rather than preconception. As the exercise unfolds, become aware of judgments: liking and moving toward what you perceive as pleasant and resisting what you do not like and perceive as unpleasant. As human beings, we all judge. Be careful not to judge the judging and simply be aware of it. Reactivity can sap our energy and rob us of a feeling of acceptance, of feeling okay with what is, even when we don't like it. Rather than letting them consume us, we open to an engaged relationship with our difficult emotions.

As you move through the exercise, notice whether you are resisting or responding. Practice allowing your process to be exactly as it is right now. We are cultivating an attitude of self-compassion, kind awareness of being with things as they are. Resisting and pushing away unpleasant emotions, sensations, and thoughts adds to the unpleasant experience. We are practicing friendliness toward all experience, in each moment. Like scientists, we are learning about our way of being in the laboratory of life, shining a spotlight on our habits to become aware of how we engage in each moment.

Often, we may become aware for the first time how preferences keep us in a habituated, reactive dance. As you engage genuine expression, you may find that you begin to let go of needing approval or direction. Trust your inner guidance.

Find a comfortable position, either on the floor or at a table, and place the sheet of paper in front of you. Begin by making a mark—any mark—anywhere on your paper and then continue mark-making in a free and playful way. Make marks of different widths; different shades; and different consistencies, shapes, and forms—for example, a hard edge versus a smudgy or soft edge. Explore light versus dark, soft versus hard, large versus small, overlapping versus parallel, solo versus multiple, spaced out versus crowded, sharp edges versus curvy lines. Express whatever marks you want with a sense of curiosity, imagination, and wonder.

Create a visual expression, letting a conversation emerge, mark by mark, on the page. There is no plan, no goal, and no preconceived idea. You are simply creating a visual expression of who you are in this moment.

Stay open to risk and surprise, following the thread one mark at a time. This process requires presence in each moment, engaging a quality of aliveness. Let go of all past experience and stand in the process of now.

When you finish, put your materials down, close your eyes, and take three deep breaths. What are you feeling? Where are you feeling sensation in the body? What emotions are present? What thoughts are you experiencing? Open your eyes and begin writing.

_____

_____

_____

_____

_____

Looking at your completed drawing, observe the shapes, lines, forms, and different media that you have chosen and how they relate. What do you see? What emotions are bubbling up? What sensations? What thoughts?

_____

_____

_____

Bring awareness to your response as you look. Is judgment present? Most of us have a harsh inner critic. Are you judging yourself harshly? Are you familiar with the judging voice?

_____

_____

_____

_____

Any time you repeat this exercise, journal about your experience.

Mindful Art Encounter #7: Letting Go

Material: Your drawing from Mindful Art Encounter #6, pen or pencil, journal

Begin by closing your eyes and recalling a time when you felt a sense of loss, perhaps the breakup of a relationship, the loss of a job, financial loss, illness, or the death of a loved one. How are you feeling it in your body, and what is your relationship to loss? Are you resisting it? Or letting it be?

Retrieve the drawing you did in Mindful Art Encounter #6. Now, rip up the drawing. Rip and tear that neat shape of paper into as many pieces as you wish, feeling into the process of ripping the paper. How does this feel? What are the sensations in your body? What are your emotions? What are your thoughts?

Notice your emotions and sensations as you are given the instruction to rip up your drawing. Is there resistance? Sadness? Anger? A feeling of loss and wanting to save this thing that you have so carefully created? Or is there a sense of surprise, surrender, and an opening to new possibility? There may be a feeling of wild abandon and excitement, a freedom of letting it be and not holding so tightly to what you hold precious and dear. A feeling of reclaiming your life and meeting fear with courage. What feelings are you aware of as you continue ripping and as the drawing becomes less and less recognizable?

When you finish ripping, put all the pieces down. Close your eyes. Take three deep breaths and feel what is to be felt in the body. As you begin to accept the experience as it is, inquire into this moment of inviting spaciousness or allowing, and seeing things as they are. Be fully present, aware, and awake. What thoughts, feelings, and sensations are you experiencing now? Experience them all. Notice any judgments, resistance and allow the experience to be exactly as it is. There is no need to change anything.

Open your eyes. Do you see anything new? As you observe the torn pieces, how do you feel?

- Are you experiencing a sense of loss, sadness, or not knowing what to do next?

- Can you hang out with the feeling of not knowing what to do?

- Can you become okay with pausing instead of quickly jumping in to fix, change, and solve?

- Can you feel into your vulnerability? Into your loss of control?

_____

_____

_____

_____

_____

Begin to move the pieces around and play with their relationships to one another. How many ways can you move them around? Try placing them overlapping, close to each other, far apart, interwoven, joined, grouped, clustered, parallel, angled, diagonal, vertical, horizontal, tightly connected, with some folded to create three-dimensional forms, falling off the page, hidden, revealed, simplified, divided, united, with space in between. Play with the idea that the pieces are not fixed and can be moved around and put in different positions. Experiment. When you're finished, set the pieces aside in a safe place.

Any time you repeat this exercise, journal about your new experience.

Mindful Art Encounter #8: Rebuilding, Collage Part 1

Materials: Torn drawing from Mindful Art Encounter #7, paper, glue, pen or pencil, journal

Start by taking three deep breaths, feeling the inhalation and exhalation and the sensations of breath in the body.

Observe the different shapes of the torn pieces of paper from the previous exercise, noticing where the torn edges are jagged and smooth. Do the torn pieces evoke any feelings?

Glue the torn pieces onto a new piece of paper, positioning them in a new way. Begin to see how, moment to moment, the pieces form a new relationship to each other and to the paper as they come together to form a new composition. By moving pieces around, you can change the shapes of the spaces between the shapes—the negative space, which can itself become interesting and take the collage in a new direction.

Notice the unexpected chance occurrence. Explore relationships as you glue, placing pieces parallel, overlapping, coming off the edge, grouped together and separate, touching, close, or apart.

What are you beginning to see? Are there any surprises or fresh inspirations? Slowly let go of the old creation as it begins to fade into the past. Stand in the present, fully engaged and awake to inspiration, new ideas, and a new perception of the earlier destruction to see more clearly the possibilities right now. Open your palms wide, allowing room for creativity and innovation, rather than holding tightly with closed fists onto what was there before. Are you feeling alive in this moment? Or are you holding onto the past and feeling a sense of regret, wanting to go back to what was?

Any time you do this exercise, journal about your experience.

Mindful Art Encounter #9: Opening to Your Reality

Materials: Your collage from Mindful Art Encounter #8, paper, glue, pencils, markers, and assorted art materials, pen or pencil, journal

Observe the collage you made in the last exercise and open your observation further. How can you add lines, shapes, and forms to connect parts of the drawing in new ways? Using whatever art materials inspire you, add lines in black or colors to form a thread that runs through the new composition. You may want to add dots of different sizes or colors, shapes of different sizes and colors, or maybe even draw over some of the new shapes to form even newer shapes. It is a conversation that keeps on unfolding moment to moment.

Try adding additional torn pieces to create a different dynamic. The process of collage is alive. The pieces that are glued down form new relationships to one another. In addition, notice a three-dimensional element forming where some of the edges reach away from the surface and become sculptural.

The spaces between objects have so much to say. Notice what you see in the empty spaces between the glued-down pieces. Are you inspired to add to these spaces or comfortable with leaving them empty? Edges, too, have so much to say. What have you learned about your own personal edge? What is the shape of your edge? How do you feel when invited to move to your edge?

As you play, step back and observe what is happening and become aware of your awareness. Seeing things from a wider view can shed light on your resistance, self-talk, and desire to control. It can show you how your perception colors your life. Remember, there are no mistakes. If you do something that you do not like after it has been created, breathe into it and see what can be created out of the thing that you do not like. It is a work in progress, with engaged presence in each moment. Ask yourself: What if I do this? What if I do that? The process becomes like a dance of listening deeply and creating from this place. Close your eyes and feel into the experience.

Keep going until you feel the conversation is complete in a new way. Are you surprised by the result? By not having had a specific plan? By simply responding to the call: "What is next?"

As you come to the end of the exercise, put your materials down and breathe in this moment, bringing awareness to your breath, body, sensations, and emotions. What have you observed about your process? Write about it below, considering the following questions:

- What is your relationship to edges? To endings? To risk? To loss? To trusting your inner guidance? To change? To new beginnings? To starting over?

  _____

  _____

  _____

  _____

- What about your relationship to silence? Freedom? Spaciousness? To saying no? To kindness? To self compassion?

  _____

  _____

  _____

  _____

Any time you do this exercise, journal about your experience.

REFLECTING ON THE WEEK

When you finish the week's work, take some time to reflect before going on. Write in your journal or on the blank lines on whichever of the reflections or prompts below speak to you.

Reflections

- Perception colors our lives. Many of us are engaged in an incessant thinking process—judging, regretting the past, hoping for the future—dictated by habits and expectations that keep us stuck in a dance of preferences and evaluations, always wishing for another "now," rather than being open to experiencing the moment as it is.

- Freedom comes from seeing things as they are, without a need to fix or change. By introducing open awareness, curiosity, and acceptance, you can experience life more freely and joyfully.

- The breath is a reliable, ever-present process that you can return your attention to again and again as an anchor to the present moment, the *nowscape* in which you are aware of your body, your breath, your emotions, and the creative voice within.

Journal Prompts

This week has been about deepening your understanding of your inner dialogue. Are you your own best friend: kind and supportive? Or do you speak to yourself with a voice full of judgment, opinions, controls, and manipulations?

Take a few minutes to journal about your inner dialogue and how it relates to circumstances in your life, answering the following questions:

- What is your inner conversation? Do you speak kindly or harshly to yourself?

- When difficulties arise and things fall apart, how do you find resources to draw upon such as kindness, courage, imagination, support, care, love, and self-compassion?

- When you need to rebuild, are you able to draw on patience, understanding, gentleness, and encouragement?

- When you need to recalibrate, are you able to draw on inner strength, resilience, and vulnerability and trust that you will learn and transform?

_____

_____

_____

_____

_____

_____

Write down your reflections on this week. What have you learned about yourself? Any ahas? What have you learned about your relationship to yourself and to others, to change? To surprise, to spontaneity, and to experimentation and curiosity? To trusting your inner guidance?

_____

_____

_____

How will this new perspective inform your life going forward? What is it that you need to invite into your daily practice? What would you like to let go of? Can you bring to mind a particular experience where you may have been unkind and judgmental? How can you experiment with a different, kinder attitude—and how might this make you feel?

_____

_____

_____

What did you learn about your experience that you particularly want to remember?

_____

_____

After you have written, close your eyes and notice the sensations in your body, emotions, and thoughts.

Week 3

Being Present

Ask yourself from time to time, "Am I awake now?" Wherever you go, there you are.

—Jon Kabat-Zinn, *Wherever You Go, There You Are*

We all engage with life uniquely, yet we are also interconnected—not only through the air we share, but also through our sensations and thoughts. And when we each share our stories, we realize that we *all* experience challenges, albeit in different ways. You are not alone in your experience.

Early in our lives, we learn how to please others—living by their values, not being able to say no, wanting to impress them—all the while hiding behind a mask, afraid to show our true nature. Eventually, we become so comfortable with the experience of hiding that this becomes our familiar way of being in the world. Habits of speech, attitudes of negativity and positivity, our inner dialogue and dialogue with others, judgments of self and others—so much time is spent in fixed ideas and automatic pilot, rather than in the experience of the moment. How often do you become lost in thought, either remembering and rehashing the past or projecting, planning, and hoping for the future, causing you to miss the precious experience of *now* as you rush toward your goals? The constant tug-of-war between moving away and resisting what we find unpleasant and moving toward what we find pleasant keeps us always *wanting* rather than accepting what is.

What if, instead, you began to slow down and relax your tight-fisted, white-knuckled hold on life? What if you held life softly and gently with humble acceptance, opening the palms of your hands to receive whatever comes—the pleasant, the unpleasant, and everything that is more neutral for you? What if you were to give thanks for *all* experience life has to offer, even when it is unexpected, unwanted, and unpleasant knowing that these categories may shift with hindsight?

When we release our grip on needing things to be a certain way—our need to control—we begin to inhabit the present moment, tasting a new engagement with our lives. Authenticity begins to shine through the cracks as we take off the mask and stand in our truth without apology or excuses. We stand in our own skin, reborn. We become curious, investigating life as if it were a scientific experiment, learning from direct experience.

The "No" Practice

For many of us, modern life involves so many voices tugging at our lives: friends and family asking for help; emails shouting, "Read me! This is important!"; articles plying us with information so we can have more, learn more, achieve more; opportunities that shouldn't be missed. We are bombarded by sounds, information, advertisements, technology, societal expectations.

Learning to say no—and to say it with clarity and conviction—is difficult, yet it is one of the most important and powerful practices. If we are busy saying yes to more than we can handle, how can we appreciate the moment? We are too busy rushing to the next moment on the treadmill, pleasing and doing, not wanting to let anyone down. But giving from a place of depletion is not healthy or mindful. It does not serve the world.

From a young age, I loved spacious blocks of quiet time—I could choose to fill them or to simply daydream and engage with each moment, without doing or planning anything. Now, as an adult, I am discerning about what I say yes to. Rather than simply filling time to distract, I let intention guide my choices. Whom do you invite into

Authentic experience is filled with acceptance, trust in one's true nature, faith, and presence. Fully awake, aware, and alive in the moment, we begin to understand the difference between how life *ought* to be and how life actually *is* as we engage with our senses to taste, touch, see, hear, and feel sensations and emotions. We befriend the stranger who has been with us all the while. We come back to our home, celebrating love from within, aligned fully with our core values and accepting of *all* experience—not only joy but also anger, fear, resentment, jealously, detachment, and sadness as a part of being alive.

One of the most important tools in your journey is the sitting meditation practice, designed to bring greater awareness to the present moment as you bring your attention to the breath. Your breath is with you for life, always present, connecting you to your body, and you can access it any time without having to do anything. As you attend to your breath and fully experience the rhythm and the process of your breathing, moment to moment, you may become more familiar with the particular rhythm of your inhalations and exhalations. Connecting with your breath invites you to be present for all experience: eating, tasting, seeing, touching, smelling, and the richness of sensing and feeling the ever-changing moments all around you.

When you practice sitting and connecting to your breath with regularity, you are learning to be with yourself. You connect to your intuition, recognizing an inner voice, and invite it in to share its wisdom. You become aware of the feeling of holding back, of not living authentically, and thus not genuinely engaging with your life. You begin to see areas where you're hiding behind the mask of conforming, pleasing, expectations, judgments, and fear.

As you let go of control and the need to fit in, you begin to freely and naturally open up to yourself and your direct experience, rather than living through other people's ideas and expectations. You can surrender to what is, without needing to change things. No more a victim of circumstance, you now may begin to see that all circumstances are workable.

As you take off the mask of unawareness, you invite your true self to the party of self-discovery. *Vulnerability* arises from acknowledging your fears. You can learn to work with your fear, letting the fear be present rather than resisting it or trying to change or ignore it. Once you are aware of your preconceived ideas and perceptions about fear, you can choose to relate differently. You can now step into your true nature, with all of its nuances—which are no longer judged as such but are simply embraced as part of who you are. With engaged curiosity and new learning, you become aware of *choice* in how you respond, rather than reacting in old worn-out ways.

Strengthened with this new awareness, you can begin to mine the jewels of your true nature, opening doorways to newly discovered hidden rooms of shame, denial, and dark experiences. Look into these new spaces with curiosity. Some rooms have glowing morning light streaming in from the windows; other rooms are darker, but as you acclimate to the darkness, you can begin to quietly and introspectively explore the shadows and light. Rather than rejecting what you do not want to see, familiarize yourself with kind acceptance. Each room is different, with its own mood and light, transforming from moment to moment. Accept all of these rooms into your home: the home of being, your true nature.

Making friends with vulnerability requires building the muscles behind your core values. We begin to talk to ourselves with a new voice—a voice of kindness and self-compassion—as we become aware of the harsh voice that beats us up. Let the harsh voice know that you are aware of its bullying and ask it to stop. *Quiet down.*

You are becoming aware of the box you have created with judgments, preferences, and perceptions and how

your circle? How do you nourish your body? What do you expose yourself to? What we take into our life experience affects us deeply.

Saying no can offer you freedom, space to be quiet, space to *be*. Saying no is a radical act of self-love, kind attention, compassion, and self-care. It is a daily practice that can feel uncomfortable and difficult at first and becomes easier with time. It then becomes a celebration and affirmation for your life. As you learn to say no, you befriend the love that is within, which is loving and accepting yourself without needing approval, achievements, or accolades from others. There is no greater gift than to say a present "no" that is clear without guilt or a longing to be loved.

In saying no, we invite space and silence into our lives. Silence invites us to drop down beneath words, ideas, chatter, and concepts to listen to our heart's longing, to shake up assumptions about ourselves, our habits, and our complacency about the way we live our lives.

In spacious silence, you may experience clarity, peace, and meaning. Then, when you do say yes, it is from the heart of good intention.

this box has kept your true nature hidden. This bully box needs to fall apart. Let's bring down the walls and open the door! *Now* begins a new journey of exploration. Let's build a new reality from the ground up, with a solid foundation of intention, attention, and awareness and using bricks of friendliness, creativity, kindness, love, acceptance, authenticity, vulnerability, honesty, direct experience, trust, curiosity, and courage. Self-compassion, presence, and acceptance bring us to the fullness of life—with all of its colors, dimensions, and nuanced experiences. Here we stop sleepwalking through life and awaken to the miracle of *now*.

Caretake this moment.

Immerse yourself in its particulars. Respond to this person, this challenge, this deed.

Quit the evasions. Stop giving yourself needless trouble.

It is time to really live; to fully inhabit the situation you happen to be in now. You are not some disinterested bystander. Participate. Exert yourself.

Respect your partnership with providence. Ask yourself often: How may I perform this particular deed such that it would be consistent with and acceptable to the divine will? Heed the answer and get to work.

When your doors are shut and your room is dark, you are not alone. The will of nature is within you as your natural genius is within. Listen to its importunings. Follow its directives.

As concerns the art of living, the material is your own life. No great thing is created suddenly. There must be time.

Give your best and always be kind.

—Epictetus

WEEK 3 INTENTIONS

During this week of the MBSE program, you may begin:

- To experience the pleasure and power of being present.

- To let go of old patterns and open space in your life for possibility, surprise, courage, and risk, knowing that you learn from *all* experience, not only what you prefer.

- To allow in vulnerability and accept yourself as you truly are.

- To practice saying "yes" and "no" with clarity and intention, rather than guilt or a longing to be loved.

WEEK 3 DAILY PRACTICE

The list below details your practice for week 3. Read through it and, if you like, use it to prepare in advance for the week's practice. You can download a printable version of this list at http://www.newharbinger.com/44932 and post it in a place where you can see it easily. Visit the same URL to download the Art of Mindfulness Practice Guide, which contains directions for the body scan, sitting meditation, and gentle stretching yoga. Audio guides for these practices are available there, too, as are printable files of the Pleasant and Unpleasant Events calendars and the Record of Mindful Moments (these can also be found at the back of this book).

1. Every day, try one of the week 3 Mindful Art Encounters in the sections that follow.

2. Alternate between doing a body scan meditation and gentle stretching yoga each day. Write in your journal, making note of anything that comes up during the exercises.

3. Practice sitting meditation for ten minutes per day.

4. Continue adding one entry per day to the Pleasant Events and Unpleasant Events calendars.

5. Continue bringing mindfulness to routine activities and record your thoughts in the Record of Mindful Moments.

6. Become aware of following the "No" Practice. If you feel the urge to say yes, pause and take three deep breaths before responding.

7. Continue writing your daily gratitude list. Each morning, write down five things you are grateful for as you begin the day. Then, in the evening as you recall your day, list five more things.

8. Complete the Reflecting on the Week section at the end of this chapter.

Mindful Art Encounter #10: Taking Off the Mask

Materials: Two pieces of paper, pencil, markers, crayons, scissors, pen or pencil, journal

Note: Before starting this exercise, review the guide for the improvisational movement meditation found in the Art of Mindfulness Practice Guide found at http://www.newharbinger.com/44932.

For thousands of years, people from many traditions have made masks to tap into inner resources, emotions, and feelings. Masks have been used in rituals and to enact characters, celebrate holidays, tell stories, and empower. This art encounter is designed to touch on the power of vulnerability, showing us how taking off the mask we hide behind brings us home to our true nature and the heart of humanity that we all share.

Mindfulness is about being genuine, authentic, celebrating our connection to life and to one another in each moment. Taking off one's mask is a radical act of acceptance and self-compassion, kindness, and inner power. It is the act of stepping into our lives fully, affirming our place in the world, and standing firm in that which we are: alive and a precious spark of humanity.

Part 1: Mask-Making

To begin this encounter, take a moment to become aware of who you are in this moment in your life. Take a few deep breaths and become present. Notice what thoughts, feelings, and sensations are present.

Take a piece of paper and place it against your face. Press it down and feel the shape around your nose and the position of your eyes. Crease and pinch the paper to mark your nose and the position of your eyes. Now, look at the paper and use the slight marks as guides to make a mask. You might want to pierce holes in the paper where the eyes are so you can see and make a slit for your mouth.

Place this paper with the slight echo of a face in front of you. Choose crayons in whatever colors you want to express your mask-self. Begin to draw on your blank mask to represent yourself right now. You may be feeling shy, doubtful, stuck, joyful, excited, afraid—be real with all that you are experiencing. Whatever it is, represent it on the mask. Have fun with it. How does your mask convey you? As in the conversation drawing, make lines, shapes, and forms to express the feelings and emotions present in your mask-self. What colors will you use for each emotion and sensation? Notice how particular colors align with particular sensations and emotions and how thoughts may inspire colors, too.

If words come to mind, include them in the overall expression of your mask-self while noticing your wanting to use words and how language sometimes drowns out feelings. We are born with two forms of expression: verbal and nonverbal. We often ignore the nonverbal and rely on the verbal, but words alone do not suffice. Use this exercise as a means to *feel* the experience rather than describe it. Feel into the possibility that one word or phrase incorporated into the drawing may be a strong addition. Stay as engaged as possible in the feelings, sensations, and emotions as you draw. Express whispers, shouts, screams, songs, or poems—whatever you feel inspired to express. Express your "mask" as clearly and directly as you can.

When you have finished, put the crayons down and close your eyes. Take a deep breath and feel into the sensation of what this mask-self is communicating to you. Allow the thoughts and feelings represented in the mask to be present. Now put on the mask and notice how you feel.

Look inside yourself—into the attic and basement and all places where things could be hidden—using courage and care. After acknowledging these well-hidden places, set the intention to clean out anything that can be let go of, anything holding you back and keeping you from fully experiencing all of your life. Call on kind self-awareness, discovering and witnessing your life as if from a bird's-eye view. This awareness without attachment can bring new insight. There is no need to hide, change, or fix. With courage and an open heart, be willing to see things clearly and step into your life fully so you can begin to breathe into each moment and reclaim your birthright of being alive and able to create.

Take a few minutes to write about this experience in your journal, using whichever of the following prompts speak to you:

- Does wearing a mask keep you feeling safe and comfortable?

- What is your biggest fear? How does this scare you? Where do you feel the fear in your body? List ways that you are hiding behind the mask-self. What quality are you ashamed of? What do you think will happen if you reveal this quality to the world?

- Do you wear the mask in your relationships, at work, or just showing up in the world?

- Is the mask about feeling stuck or not good enough? If so, what are you afraid of? What is holding you back?

- What is your relationship to being fully present? Can you recall moments of presence?

- What is your relationship to joy and happiness? What is the difference between joy and happiness? Do you feel that you deserve to be happy? What brings you joy?

- What is your relationship to sadness? How does sadness feel? Where do you feel it in your body, and what are the sensations?

- What is your relationship to anger? What is the felt sense? Does anger have a shape? How do sensations of anger show up in your body?

- Are there parts of you that feel shame? What does shame feel like? How do you experience feeling shame?

- When you look at your mask, what do you see? Are you surprised by the rendering?

- Is there judgment of how your mask looks? For example, were you bothered that the marks for the eyes and nose were amorphous and not symmetrical? Are these judgments connected to other areas of your life? Is this judgment familiar?

- What does perfectionism mean to you? Are you striving to be perfect in any area of your life? How does this striving affect your being?

Put on your mask and begin to move, following the improvisational movement meditation guide. Feel into the authenticity and wisdom of the body, expressing the form and content of your drawing through original, imaginative movement and rhythms. Listen to your body and how it wants to move, echoing the energy of the mask. You can move to music or in silence.

As you wind down, take a moment to see what comes up for you as you prepare to take off your mask. Notice the sensations you feel in your body. What energy is present? How is the quality of your breath?

Now take off your mask. Who are you without your mask? Notice what you are feeling. Is there any judgment? Invite kindness and safety to allow for vulnerability so your true nature can shine through. What are you revealing now without your mask on? Is there fear? There may also be elation, freedom, relief, and deep appreciation. What are you willing to invite in without your mask? Notice what insights you have. Can you live into the question: Who am I without my mask?

How are you feeling after this exercise? Participants often have a feeling of sadness as they recognize—sometimes for the first time—how much energy has been invested in hiding behind a mask.

Rest in this moment of seeing, thinking, feeling, and sensing. What will you do with this one precious life? Will you be brave and live authentically? Can you live from the inside out, rather than from the external expectations of society, family, and relationships and the inner expectations that you demand of yourself?

Walk around in silence and feel the sensations in your body. Feel emotions and bring awareness to your thoughts. Feel the authenticity bubbling up and whether you are accepting of this unmasked version of a self that may be longing to emerge as a free and creative spirit.

To have patience with everything unsolved in your heart and try to love the questions themselves as if they were locked rooms or books written in a very foreign language. Don't search for the answers, which could not be given to you now, because you would not be able to live them. And the point is to live everything. Live the questions now. Perhaps, then, some day far in the future, you will gradually, without even noticing it, live your way into the answer.

—Rainer Maria Rilke, *Letters to a Young Poet*, translated by Stephen Mitchell

Part 2: Unmasking

Now rip up your mask, feeling the sensations as your hands and arms tear it apart, one piece at a time. Are you ripping quickly or slowly? Carefully or forcefully? Sadly or angrily? Gently or powerfully? Aggressively or kindly? Breathe into what you are feeling as you rip up your mask.

Pause. Take three deep breaths and observe the torn pieces. Feel into what they represent. What is bubbling up for you as you look at the pieces? What do you see?

After you have looked and allowed what you saw to be felt, begin to reassemble the pieces in a new way, with the intention of discarding the pieces that no longer serve you. How can you reveal your true, boundless face?

Remember, there is no right or wrong way to do this. There is only the invitation to listen deeply to whatever needs to be expressed right now. When we slow down, the act of observing deepens into looking as we pause and see with our eyes and heart and with full awareness of the emotions and sensations in the body.

Which pieces need to be included? How shall the pieces be glued together to create a new face of acceptance and kindness? This is the face of your true nature. The mask is off, revealing a genuine and vulnerable self. This includes *all* the aspects of self, including those that may not be pretty, that you may have disowned: your shadow self. This new face welcomes all aspects—all parts of you—with kindness and without judgment. This is the face of accepting who you are.

Now how about adding color? What lenses do you see the world through?

No matter what the lenses or the color, being vulnerable is the first step to opening up and inviting a new way of seeing and being: no longer fixed and solid, but spacious, curious, and open-hearted with a beginner's mind that is free, open, and engaged. By embodying different lenses and colors, we can re-create our reality from a more mindful, aware perspective of being the seer and the seen.

Any time you do this exercise, journal about your experience.

Mindful Art Encounter #11: Accepting

Materials: Blindfold (optional), paper, pencil, markers, glue, eraser, crayons, journal

Note: Before starting this exercise, review the guide for sitting meditation found in the downloadable Art of Mindfulness Practice Guide found at http://www.newharbinger.com/44932.

Start this exercise with a five-minute sitting meditation. Just "be" with all of the experience.

When you have finished, place your paper in front of you and your art materials within reach. Close your eyes or use a blindfold so you cannot see the marks as you make them. Place the pencil, markers, or crayons in your nondominant hand and begin to express the feeling of not being in control, of vulnerability, on the paper. Start with a line and then continue with adding lines, shapes, marks, and dots—all intuitive expressions of the feeling of being vulnerable as you make marks without the usual control of your steadier hand.

With this experience of not seeing and drawing with your nondominant hand, you are beginning to explore what it feels like to let go of your usual ways of doing and being, to get out of your comfort zone and familiar ways, and to engage with discomfort and loss of control.

Remember, there is no right or wrong way. Press as hard or softly as you want to express your vulnerability.

Take your time, feeling into the sensations in your hand as you hold the pencil or marker. How does it feel to use your nondominant hand? Is there resistance and judgment, or are you open to a new sensation of experimenting, accepting, or surprise?

How do you feel about using random colors that you pick up while blinded to seeing and choosing? What markers, thin or thick, have you felt in your hand? Can you feel the width of the lines from a thick marker, if that is what you picked up? How often have you changed materials, or have you stuck to one? As you draw, how does it feel when you make a curvy line, a straight line, or a sharp line with points? Can you feel into the line being created? What are you feeling? If you begin to feel your inner critic, notice it and then come back to the creation at hand, marking the moment of exploration, of vulnerability.

When you are finished, put down the pencil, marker, or crayon and consider the following questions, writing your answers in the lines below or in your journal.

- How did it feel to not be able to see what you were drawing?

- How did it feel to use your nondominant hand?

- How did you connect with the feeling of vulnerability?

- What did you learn about your relationship to letting go of control and your expectations and judgments about how you wanted this process to feel?

- Were you able to stay open to surprise and making a mess?

- Did your sitting practice inform this process? What was the relationship between the two?

- Was doing the drawing helpful in realizing your relationship to vulnerability and acceptance?

_____

_____

_____

_____

_____

_____

_____

_____

_____

Any time you do this exercise, journal about your experience.

Mindful Art Encounter #12: Seeing Clearly

Materials: Paper, pencils, markers, crayons, eraser, glue, journal

Note: Before starting this exercise, review the guide for walking meditation found in the downloadable Art of Mindfulness Practice Guide found at http://www.newharbinger.com/44932.

Start by doing a walking meditation for five minutes. You will thus be inviting the experience of walking mindfully to spill over onto the paper.

Imagine walking into the landscape of your being, into who you are in this moment expressed as a landscape. Tread the ground and feel the terrain and surroundings. Sense the experience of your landscape.

Notice, in the vast and precious landscape of your life, what you have learned and where you stand in this moment. As you continue to practice on a regular basis, you'll likely begin to see more clearly. You now know that you can begin again in each moment. You can choose tools—such as the body scan, sitting meditation, gentle stretching yoga, and awareness of breath meditation—to practice responding to the ever-changing landscape of your life. Choose to see your stuckness, habits, and perceptions with open acceptance. Introduce kindness so everything is workable and you are not trying to fit into a preconceived idea. Rather, engage in the experience of life happening each moment. It is a similar process to the improvisation you experienced in the conversation drawing (encounter #6). You have choices, you have tools to remind you when you forget, and you have the option to open your perspective and see the bigger picture—the vast interconnectedness of the human experience. We all experience closing, and opening to new perspectives within, the vast horizon of interconnectedness just as the in-breath expands and the out-breath contracts, in due course.

On the paper, begin to create the landscape of your life in this moment. Where is the horizon line? How much of the page is land, and how vast is your sky? What does the land represent to you? What does the sky represent? What does the horizon line represent? Is there a significant horizon line? How does vegetation appear in your landscape? What is the weather? The temperature? Are there clouds, sunshine, wind, snow? What is the season? Is it light or dark? Day or night? Can you see the ocean, or are you in the forest? Are you in a meadow, in a valley, on a mountain, in a field or cave, by the ocean, on the bank of a river, on an island? Is it scary or safe? Use the language of lines, shapes, forms, dots, broken lines, curvy lines, thick lines, thin lines, hard edges, soft edges, bold marks, and whisper strokes. Do strong, dark, deliberate lines or passive lines better express the landscape of your life now? As you begin to play with spontaneity and surprise, how does this process of improvisation feel? Is there a sense of flow and fun?

Use your imagination and choose colors that speak to your actual experience, rather than simply using blue for the sky and green or brown for the ground. For example, you might try a color that is bold and speaks of a truly personal landscape. Feel free to mix colors or use lines, shapes, and dots of different colors. It can be as simple or as intricate as you wish.

Play with the drawing to express how you feel. Stand in this moment and inhabit the ground of your being. Feel your connection to the earth: imagine roots reaching from the soles of your feet deep into the terrain and the support available to you at any moment in your landscape.

Notice what you are feeling as you create your landscape. What are you sensing? What are your emotions and thoughts? Feel into the full process of improvisation. What is being revealed to you in the making and marking?

After you have expressed this visual landscape of your life, put your materials down. Close your eyes. Pause; take three deep breaths. Stay open to the messages and whispers in the moment.

How did this experience feel in your body? What insights have you had? How have you crossed your landscape? Write your answer without thinking too much about it.

_____

_____

_____

_____

_____

Now draw a dot or a shape, large or small, in any position in the landscape. This indicates your relationship to the ground, the horizon, and the sky. You can color this dot or shape however you wish. Is the shape large or small? Is it rooted to the ground or flying in the sky? Use your imagination. Be spontaneous. What is your shape: circle, square, vertical line? Is it solid or only an outline? Does your shape touch the horizon? Is it between ground and sky, crossing the horizon? How were you inspired to place your shape? What is your sense of relating to others in your life? Where are they in the landscape of the life that you share? Are there defining lines that separate you from them? Is there a sense of interconnecting where the lines that separate us dissolve into shared experiences?

Any time you repeat this exercise, journal about your experience.

Mindful Art Encounter #13: Self-Portrait: Seeing Things as They Are

Materials: Paper, pencils, markers, crayons, eraser, glue, journal

You have been practicing several of the most important formal mindfulness tools in our journey inward: the body scan, sitting meditation, awareness of breath meditation, mindful eating, and walking meditation. Each of these tools is designed to bring greater awareness of engaging with the present moment. For example, in sitting meditation, we practice bringing our attention to body sensations, breath, sounds, and choiceless awareness. In awareness of breath meditation, we focus on the breath and the process of inhalation and exhalation and then the breath in the body. In the body scan, we bring attention to sensations in the body together with the process of breath in the body as it receives and releases air. Walking meditation focuses on sensations of the body in motion, with all of our muscles engaged. And in mindful eating, we use sound, sight, touch, smell, and taste sensations to experience eating.

Select a practice you would like to do before this exercise, referring to the online guide if necessary. Your choice is important. You are likely beginning to realize which practices feel most beneficial to you in the moment; design your practice accordingly.

After you have finished your practice, create an abstract drawing as a self-portrait using whatever art materials best express the qualities of your experience in this moment when you see things as they are. Use pencils, markers, and crayons to draw colors, lines, shapes, and forms. Avoid words and symbols. What colors express your experience now? What is the essence: lines, dots, patterns, overlapping shapes, textures?

What kind of composition are you creating? Are the marks and lines filling the space, or are there open spaces? What does this process feel like in your body? Are there sensations or emotions? Do some marks capture the busy thoughts in your head, judgments, or needing things your way, versus the quiet moments of attending to your breath and feeling creative flow living through you? There is no right or wrong way to do this exercise. With childlike curiosity, play with your imagination and improvisation, without any expectations for the end result. Experiment without preconceived ideas of how you want it to look.

When you are finished, pause and observe your drawing. Look back at the body scan self-portrait you created in week 1. Consider the following questions and then write the answers below or in your journal:

- How is this self-portrait different?

- How has your understanding changed?

- Does this abstract self-portrait feel as if it holds within it a playful record of the moment?

- Did the formal mindfulness practice inspire your creative process, and how were they connected?

- How did the practice spill over into the creative process?

- Was it helpful to begin the encounter with a formal practice of your choice?

- Were you aware of thoughts? Did you experience moments of engagement in the drawing process?

- Have you become aware of patterns and habits? Is your experience of self changing in any way? How?

_____

_____

_____

_____

_____

_____

_____

_____

Sit with these questions and see what bubbles up for you. Be present with all that is felt, sensed, and thought as it is in the moment. Notice whether your self-talk is kind or harsh. If you'd like, journal about your experience. Use words, doodles, scribbles, or other visual means.

Any time you repeat this exercise, journal about your experience.

REFLECTING ON THE WEEK

When you finish the week's work, take some time to reflect before going on. Write in your journal or on the blank lines on whichever of the reflections or prompts below speak to you.

Reflections

- By allowing yourself to be vulnerable, you can take off your mask and live your authentic life, which is the only way to live fully in the present moment.

- Immersing in the present is a gift you can give yourself and the world, learning to differentiate between your *thoughts* about something and the actual direct experience of sensations and emotions. Your body is the doorway to tasting life fully.

- Learning to say no with clarity and conviction is one of the most important and powerful practices, allowing you the space and silence to listen to your heart's longing and find peace and meaning.

- Genuine creative expression is alive, authentic, and requires nothing less than an intention to become intimate with your life, to pay full attention to your body and your breath, and to be aware and awake in your life.

Journal Prompts

Write down your reflections on this week, using your journal if you need more space to write.

What have you learned about your inner dialogue and your relationship to spontaneity, improvisation, and experimentation?

_____

_____

_____

_____

_____

_____

Have you practiced saying no? Is it becoming easier? How do you feel when you have answered honestly rather than from a feeling of guilt or expectation?

_____

_____

_____

_____

_____

How will this new perspective inform your life going forward? What would you like to invite into your daily practice? What would you like to let go of?

_____

_____

_____

_____

_____

What did you learn about your experience that you particularly want to remember?

_____

_____

_____

_____

_____

After you have written, close your eyes and notice the sensations in your body, emotions, and thoughts.

Week 4

Playing

Man is most nearly himself when he achieves the seriousness of a child at play.

—Heraclitus, 535–475 BCE

The only way to truly understand the power of play is though the senses and the freedom of playful engagement. The art encounters in this chapter—and workbook as a whole—offer a doorway into the process of play.

In many ways, this week is the heart of the MBSE program, which aims to boldly inspire curiosity, joy, self-compassion, and kind attention through creative discovery of an ever-changing self that is immeasurable, incomprehensible, and indescribable. Vast and filled with creative engagement, playful improvisation and abstract exploration are like a playground, a rehearsal for living with a sense of gratitude accepting what we want with the same gracious awareness as that which we do not want.

Week 4 is thus an important lesson. It is about play, the essence of engaging with life. Your invitation for this week is to return to the child you once were: spontaneous, open, and honest. For most of us, this was a time of being curious.

As adults age, we disengage from the peculiarities of each passing moment, and we often lose the sense of spontaneous play and wonder. You may have already begun to see how your unique perceptions keep you in the groove of familiar habit that often cause you suffering. You might feel afraid of trying new ways of being in the world, of taking risks and making mistakes. Most of us want security and control, and the fear of losing those things stops the process of playful discovery.

Play is vital to engaging with life as it unfolds moment to moment with experiences and events over which we have no control. Iniviting play into your day can ease stress and help you engage with whatever arises with a sense of curious improvisation. Play is not transactional or future-focused. There is no expectation of results; the pressure is off. It gets you out of the mindset of pushing, judging, striving, competing, and producing.

Play is about immersing and responding in the moment. As children play, they respond to surprises with curiosity and wonder. They become fully immersed in the experience of *now*, feeling the sensation of experience rather than thinking about the concept of experience. The energy of play is spontaneous, without filters, preferences, or aversions. To play is to experiment, not knowing what you are doing, risking making a mess and feeling like a failure. It is about being in the process without a fixed idea of product, open to whatever happens. In fact, throughout history, play has led to many inventions and discoveries.

Through play, you can practice coming to the edge of the familiar and jumping off, trusting that you will be safely directed to new horizons, perspectives, and possibilities. This is how we transform, grow, and learn. And once you learn this through play, you will be able to bring this into your experiences of life.

Play is the process by which we understand ourselves, feel alive, and accept who we are *right now*. It requires embracing *all* of your experience with mindful curiosity, including the experiences you would rather reject. In the beginning, this may not feel like play. As you deepen your practice and bring more kindness into the process, it will become easier to let go of judgments and wanting things to be different. For example, this might mean letting go of:

> *fixed ideas, stories, control, power, stuck habits, familiar patterns, hoping to be perfect, wanting approval, fitting in, judgments, separation, feeling superior, never feeling good enough, always trying to improve, persistence, exhaustion, conforming to societal expectations, not wanting to stand out, not wanting to make waves or upset others, or avoiding voicing your resistance.*

Whenever you become aware of judging yourself harshly, take three deep breaths and get right back into playful exploration. Become aware of fears that are keeping you stuck. Engage with risk and become curious about the process, rather than the product. Invite surprise. Let go of control over how you *should* feel. Instead, infuse the knowledge you gain about yourself through play with kindness and self-compassion, affirming your place in the world.

When loss, disappointment, difficulties, and mistakes happen, you may find that you can let go of expectations and reactivity, responding and playing even when experiences are not what you like or want. You may notice being able to go with the flow, to take yourself a little less seriously. This is play with a capital P. In this way, we may discover that we become more accepting and grateful for each moment of being alive in all of its manifestations, shapes, and colors. As pediatrician and psychoanalyst Donald Winnicott said, "It is in play and only in play that the individual finds the self."

The Three-Minute Breath Space

If there is a battle going on inside you, people can feel the energy, and it is contagious. When we are more peaceful, on the other hand, we emanate a sense of calm that is felt by others. Mindful breathing is a way to feel into a sense of peace and quiet below the chatter and busyness of daily life. Breath practice nourishes your quality of being, infusing a sense of presence, calm, and kindness and easing stress, anxiety, and imbalance. It is always available and always with us; it is a simple practice that connects us to life moment to moment.

Whether it's this short, three-minute version or a longer awareness of breath meditation, use mindful breathing as a little gift of self-care, a way to stop and recharge whenever you want to ground in the present moment, away from automatic pilot.

Here's how to do the three-minute breath practice:

1. Sitting or standing comfortably, feel into your body. Feel the sensations of your buttocks being supported by the chair and your feet touching the ground.

2. Ask yourself: What is here now? Accept all that arises: thoughts, feelings, sensations, and emotions. Invite all experience in. Be present. Become aware of your breath with the curiosity of a child. Notice where you feel your breath most vividly: at the nostrils, chest, or belly? Are you breathing shallow or deeply? With long or short breaths?

3. Expand your awareness to your body as a whole.

4. Bring kind attention to everything.

Practice for three minutes. Repeat a few times during your day. You may find that it becomes a respite and a way to renew.

WEEK 4 INTENTIONS

During this week of the MBSE program, you will begin:

- To practice playful investigating, questioning, and experimentation to let go of fixed ideas and opinions, and instead dance with new rhythms and possibilities that arise in the open space of spontanous of improvisation.

- To practice infusing your life with self-compassion and kind attention.

- To practice playfully affirming your place in the world as an interdependent, interconnected living being through acts of generosity and kindness.

- To practice play as a rehearsal for letting go and embracing *all* of life's experiences.

WEEK 4 DAILY PRACTICE

The list below details your practice for week 4. Read through it and, if you like, use it to prepare in advance for the week's practice. You can download a printable version of this list at http://www.newharbinger.com/44932 and post it in a place where you can see it easily. Visit the same URL to download the Art of Mindfulness Practice Guide, which contains directions for the body scan, sitting meditation, and gentle stretching yoga. Audio guides for these practices are available there, too, as are printable files of the Pleasant and Unpleasant Events Calendars and the Record of Mindful Moments (these can also be found at the back of this book).

1. Practice one of the week 4 Mindful Art Encounters (in the sections that follow) every day.

2. Alternate the body scan with gentle stretching yoga every other day.

3. Practice a sitting meditation for ten minutes each day, paying attention to the breath and body sensations.

4. Practice mindful awareness of feeling stuck, becoming numb, and shutting off to the moment whenever it happens this week.

5. Complete the Reflecting on the Week section at the end of this chapter.

Mindful Art Encounter #14: Surprise and Play

Materials: Piece of 8½ x 11-inch paper, colored pencils and/or pens, journal

Fold a piece of paper in half and then in half again. Using only one quarter of the page, draw a feeling that is difficult for you. For example, it could be fear, anxiety, or anger. Although this may not be a quality you like, see if you can capture the essence of this quality—its energy—without judging yourself, and allow it to be present in the drawing through color, shape, line, and gesture.

Flip the paper to reveal another quarter page on the same side of the paper, now keeping only the new blank quarter-page visible. This time, think of a quality that delights you or that you are curious about, such as kindness, courage, or generosity. Bring this quality to life on the paper with color, shape, line, and gesture. See if you can connect with and express the essence of this quality.

Next, refold the paper so that only another blank quarter-page is visible on the same side of the whole page. Think of a quality that you would like to experience more of in your life, perhaps something you have been missing, such as patience, gratitude, love, vulnerability, or authenticity. Express whichever quality you chose on this quadrant with color, line, shape, and gesture.

Finally, turn the paper so the last blank quadrant on that side of the page is visible. Take a moment and reflect on mindful acceptance: mindful awareness of all the qualities that live within you. Think about the gift of acceptance and tolerance that is possible; the ability to color your reality with kind awareness, even when what you see is not easy. In this last quadrant, express mindfulness with color, line, shape, and gesture.

When you're finished, take a few deep breaths and sit quietly for a moment, and then open the page to reveal all four quadrants. Take some time to observe them. Look. Take time to engage looking. What do you notice? Does anything stand out to you? If so, write it below.

_____

_____

_____

_____

_____

Next, reflect on the connections between the four quadrants. Join the quarters by freely adding lines, shapes, and colors to integrate your experiences with the qualities of acceptance and love, representing one image of creative wholeness. How can you create a visual expression of who you are? Be free in your exploration. Have fun. Play.

Once this process is complete, set down your art materials, close your eyes, and embody the sensations and inner wisdom. Pause, breathe into the moment, and deepen curiosity and your engagement with the sensations with kind acceptance and compassion. Then, turn the paper over and write a word, phrase, or sentence that captures your experience.

Any time you do this exercise, journal about your experience.

Mindful Art Encounter #15: The Ugly Drawing

Materials: Black marker, paper, pen or pencil, journal

Note: Before starting this exercise, review the guide for the body scan found in the downloadable Art of Mindfulness Practice Guide found at http://www.newharbinger.com/44932.

One of the most important tools in our journey is the body scan, which is designed to bring greater awareness of the body in the present moment. For this art encounter, let's explore the body scan in a new way, focusing your attention on moments when your mind wanders into thoughts and stories about your body. This is an opportunity to explore your relationship to your body—your attitudes, inner dialogue, expectations, and judgments that keep you from experiencing the body directly—and how this relationship to your body colors everything in your life, including how you relate to others and the world.

Begin by noticing your inner dialogue with your body and writing about it in the lines below.

- Are any of your attitudes or beliefs keeping you from directly experiencing your body?

- What do you judge as an "ugly" part of your body?

- Pausing, bring awareness to your judging mind.

_____

_____

_____

_____

_____

_____

_____

_____

Notice how much you may expect from the body. As it is, the body is a miracle of functionalities that serves us in every moment. We rarely celebrate our bodies without wishing they were different, better, or changed in some way—perhaps more so if we are female in most societies. We have bought into messages from the media, TV, magazines, and the Internet about how we should look, about what is beautiful and what is ugly.

Most of us have harsh inner critics, causing us to worry and feel stressed, anxious, and depressed. Our conversation is often caught up in negative rather than positive thinking. We may experience low self-esteem, a negative body image, and a feeling of never being good enough—of being "ugly." This negative self-talk can keep us stuck, spilling over into health, relationships, work, and connection with the world. It can isolate and cause harm in both small and devastating ways. As you begin to practice art encounters and meditation practices, however, you can choose kindness and self-compassion to wake up, accept, and celebrate your body.

Start by sitting in a chair and doing a ten-minute body scan. As your meditation unfolds, you may feel a variety of sensations in your body—or a lack of sensation. You might also find yourself *thinking* about the body rather than feeling into the actual sensations. Thinking takes you into the judging mind. Whenever you notice judgments, it's a flag that you are thinking rather than experiencing sensations in the body. The practice is to *notice* when you are thinking. Say to yourself "thinking" and then come back to the experience of sensing in your body: seeing, hearing, tasting, touching, smelling, and thus abiding in the miracle of direct experience, of body sensations, rather than opinions and preferences.

When you are finished, notice which feelings and emotions are present. Then use a black marker to express the feeling of "ugly" on your page. Without thinking or planning what you will do, just make the first "ugly" mark. Then add to this ugly mark and make it uglier. Mark by mark and line by line, continue expressing "ugly." What types of marks or dots, straight and sharp lines, patterns and textures are you making? Press hard and jab the paper forcefully if this is what you are feeling.

Notice what you are feeling in your body as you build on the expression of ugly. As you work, consider these questions:

- Where do you feel ugly in the body?

- As you notice the inner critic raise its head and the judgment of ugly, how do you feel?

There is no right or wrong way to do this exercise. We all have a different relationship to "ugly." What one person finds ugly, another may find beautiful. Can you see your reaction to ugly? Do you find emotions ugly? Thoughts ugly? Sensations ugly? Your body ugly? Words ugly?

Drawing—as a means to investigate and experiment with relationship to aversion—can be freeing and may shine a light on the perception and sensations evoked by aversion. It may introduce a new attitude of letting go of a preference for beautiful and of judgments of ugly. There may be a new way to hold opposites in the space of acceptance and wholeness. This can inspire wakefulness and lead to kind acceptance.

It can be freeing and fun to do an "ugly" drawing, rather than trying to draw something beautiful, which may hold expectations and feel inadequate. An ugly drawing can be anything; there are no preconceived ideas or standards to live up to.

When you are finished, answer the following questions on the lines provided or in your journal.

How were the body scan and the drawing experiences related? Did one inform the other or not?

_____

_____

Were you able to observe how attached you are to having things *not* be ugly? Were you able to observe how much judgment comes into play as you evaluate what is ugly and unacceptable versus beautiful and acceptable?

_____

_____

Were you able to sense the feeling of "ugly"? What was your experience?

_____

_____

Did you feel resistance to "ugly," and if so, how did that resistance manifest (for example, as tension, discomfort, contraction, pain, or disgust)?

_____

_____

Was it helpful to draw an abstract expression of "ugly"?

_____

_____

Any time you repeat this exercise, journal about your experience.

Mindful Art Encounter #16: Destruction and Tearing Apart

Materials: Your drawing from Mindful Art Encounter #15, pen or pencil, journal

Note: Before starting this exercise, review the guide for the walking meditation found in the downloadable Art of Mindfulness Practice Guide found at http://www.newharbinger.com/44932.

Begin this exercise with a short five-minute walking meditation. As you walk, sense into the feeling of "ugly." How does this feel? Where are you experiencing this in your body?

As you feel into the experience of "ugly," with its harsh self-talk and negativity, and a feeling of not being good enough, tear up your ugly drawing from the last exercise into as many pieces as you wish. Tear up the notion of ugly! Young children see all things openly and with acceptance, while we adults have become programmed by our upbringing, environment, community, and culture to label them "beautiful" or "ugly." Can we appreciate, without the layer of evaluation? Play helps us lighten up and accept what *is*, seeing openly and spaciously that *all* things, *all* ways of being, *all* circumstances can be ugly to one person and beautiful to another. Can we rest in accepting that all is beautiful? We are beautiful exactly as we are. There is no need to change anything.

When you've finished, close your eyes and feel what is to be felt in the body. Are you feeling relief, sadness, attachment, or freedom? What are you feeling? Where are you feeling it?

_____

_____

_____

_____

_____

Pause. Take three deep breaths and sense, feel, and embody the moment as it is without trying to change anything. Just feel the raw experience. Ask yourself:

- What are your emotions?

- Where do you feel them in the body?

- Do you have thoughts that are analyzing, ruminating, projecting, regretting, or planning?

- What is the color of this moment as you breathe it all in?

_____

_____

_____

_____

_____

_____

Let's begin again with a new way of seeing the concept of "ugly." Let go of the resistance and open yourself to seeing aversion as an aspect of "beautiful," accepting all of your quirks, foibles, and challenging parts as part of the beauty of being fully alive. Accept the present without the overlay of prejudice, the inner critic, or negativity flooding in or holding tightly to your ego perspective. Can you see things as they are—not from judgments, but freshly, without bias and with the freedom of acceptance?

What is your relationship to "ugly" now? What has changed?

_____

_____

_____

_____

_____

Set your torn pieces someplace safe so you can use them for the next exercise.
Any time you repeat this exercise, journal about your experience.

Mindful Art Encounter #17: Rebuilding, Collage Part 2

Materials: Torn pieces from Mindful Art Encounter #16; colored pencils, pens, or crayons; glue; paper; journal

This art encounter is an extension of encounters #8, Rebuilding, Collage Part 1 (week 2). It invites you to open possibilities to see more deeply, revealing new options.

Start this encounter by standing in Mountain pose, another important tool in your mindfulness toolbox. This pose is designed to bring greater awareness to the body as it stands upright, anchored to the ground and filled with the strength of a mountain.

Standing with your feet hip-distance apart, arms at your sides. Stand upright with your spine straight, feeling into the body as a whole. Stay in Standing Mountain pose for three minutes. Feel the mountain breathing in and out, staying strong and connected with the air expanding and releasing the breath. Breathe into your sense of "mountain-ness": your strength and rooted presence, your dignity and uprightness.

As you become familiar with the weather of reactivity, you can learn to feel into the mountain-like quality within you. The mountain stays strong through winds, storms, floods, lightning, snow, and hurricanes. The mountain remains rooted in its mountainous quality of inner strength.

Come out of the pose and bring your attention to the torn pieces of your ugly drawing from the previous encounter. Select one piece at a time and color only *half* of the piece with a new color of love, presence, imagination, response, and acceptance and self-compassion. Continue coloring half of each piece.

Each piece of torn paper will now have two differently colored halves: one with the reactive color that feels like aversion, the other with the responding color of love.

Begin creating a new reality by gluing these pieces into a new composition, with new relationships. Before gluing the pieces into a permanent position, play with all the different possibilities.

You may choose whatever exploration you are most interested in—whether pattern, color, rhythm, or relationships of shapes and color—and follow it in-depth, improvising, playing with options and possibilities before gluing your pieces down. Like a child playing with building blocks, experiment with different creative combinations to create different structures, designs, or abstract compositions. Remember, you are in the process of the experiment that is your life. You are exploring new territory that you have not explored before. You are the only traveler of your journey; your way is different from any other. Be willing to fall down, feel lost, not know what you are doing. Keep going and commit to playing with this process of discovery. Perhaps try the following:

- Play with the notion of color.

- Place colors next to each other and see what relationships form. As you play with colors, what do you discover about colors and their placement? What does each color do to the surrounding colors? How does black relate to color? How does white relate to color?

- Play with the idea of pattern. What patterns can you come up with? How do you begin to create patterns?

- Explore the idea of rhythm, creating music though color and pattern.

- Explore how many alternate relationships can be formed. How many different ways can you find to place the torn pieces together again?

- What designs begin to form as you play?

- Play with the notion of horizontal and vertical lines, circles, or overlapping black and colored pieces to form circles, squares, triangles, or other shapes.

- Play with positive (full) and negative (empty) spaces.

Play, play, and play. As you play with all the different possibilities, feel free to take a photo of each step and inquiry. Write down the different stages of your inquiry and how the different stages and processes expanded your sense of play and possibility.

Any time you do this exercise, journal about your experience.

REFLECTING ON THE WEEK

When you finish the week's work, take some time to reflect before moving on. Write in your journal or on the blank lines on whichever of the reflections or prompts below speak to you.

Reflections

- Staying in your comfort zone is like sleepwalking though life: a way of hiding behind habits, numbing, and resisting. It is the opposite of play.

- Play involves experimentation; risk; curiosity; loosening the grip of control, fixed ideas, and expectations; and a willingness to discover new possibilities in the moment.

- Play is a way to practice and strengthen the coping skills necessary for greater ease and well-being.

- A playful approach to life leads to less stress; a more genuine, authentic acceptance of self; and the ability to love yourself as well as others.

- Play invites resilience and self-compassion.

Journal Prompts

Write down your reflections of this week. What discoveries did you make? Any ahas?

_____

_____

_____

_____

_____

_____

_____

What did you learn about play and what the process of play brings to life?

_____

_____

_____

_____

_____

Can you introduce more play into your life? Be specific. Can you be more playful in relationships? Work? Food? Exercise? What do you enjoy doing, and how can you play more in these areas?

_____

_____

_____

_____

_____

_____

_____

_____

_____

After you have written, close your eyes and notice your emotions, your thoughts, and the sensations in your body.

Accepting Wholeness

You are the drop, and the ocean.

—Jalal-al-Din Rumi, *The Essential Rumi*, translated by Coleman Barks with John Moyne

Chinese philosophy tells us there are two complimentary forces in nature, each necessary for the existence of the other. The *yin* is the softer, more receptive and nurturing force, and the *yang* is the more assertive, active force. Everything is made up of both yin and yang, and it is the interconnectedness and flow between the two that creates the energy of the whole.

Yin energy is about flexibility, receptivity, and endurance; it is inward-focused, soft, and malleable. Yang energy is more fixed, rigid, and assertive; its strength comes from being outwardly focused. Some examples of yin and yang include internal and external, inactivity and activity, stillness and movement, calm and energetic, indirect and direct, dark and light, night and day, black and white, water and fire, submissive and dominant, quiet and loud, flexible and solid, cold and hot, slow and fast, shy and bold—each part defining (and being defined by) the other.

Yin and yang may seem like opposites, but they complement each other and are in natural flow throughout our inner and outer worlds. Their interconnected energies are the unseen threads weaving the fabric of life, like an invisible web containing all living matter. It's this flowing and moving energy that creates the innate rhythms all around us and within us: patterns of breath, physical movement, wellness and healing, birth and death, day and night, light and dark, seasons, and tides. This philosophy is in direct opposition to Western thought, which has largely been centered on the dualistic hierarchy of a dominant masculine and passive feminine.

We all experience the patterns of yin and yang naturally within our bodies and lives. Our breath and all of our systems—our "beingness"—are deeply connected to the outer rhythms of others, nature, and the world around us. This way of being is effortless, only requiring that we accept and experience the fullness of each changing moment rather than trying to impose our needs, controls, expectations, and judgments. So much energy is freed up if we allow things to be as they are without needing to change or fix them. There is freedom in letting things be.

These patterns—within us and around us—transform and change in each passing moment. Nothing truly stays the same. Look around you with open attention and see the intricate patterns transforming and changing in every moment. Each morning, for example, sunrise initiates a yang cycle, the sun warming and sustaining life as people move, work, create, play, and nourish themselves. As night falls, yin energy begins. Activity slows down, and we rest, renew, and reflect. Spring and summer are active, abundant with the yang energy of flowers budding and renewed strength and light. In autumn and winter, life slows down, decays, and dies. Both yin and yang are interconnected and necessary for the life cycle, equal parts of the whole magical process.

As we experience life fully, we can bring awareness to the balance of yin and yang in our relationships, work, homes, and inner dialogue. When we are off-balance, we are reminded that something is not right. We can then choose what is needed to come back to balance. In relationships, partners take turns being receptive (yin) versus assertive (yang) to maintain harmony. In the workplace, we must spend time listening and formulating ideas (yin) as well as taking action (yang). Yin flows into yang, and yang flows into yin in the ever-changing, transformative rhythm of life. Change is constant, and so to befriend change is to embrace life fully. This is the art of living: dancing and celebrating the composition being created moment to moment.

This week, we will begin to let go and surrender to our own inner balance of yin and yang, using the art encounters as a platform for investigation. You'll learn to recognize and engage yin and yang energies within yourself and understand how their balance creates your innate gifts and affirms your unique presence in the world. Rather than fighting your natural creative energies—trying to contort and control them through resistance, judgment, and needing things to be different—you'll learn to dance with and accept this interconnectedness of yin and yang.

As you work on the art encounters in this chapter, try to recognize the forces of yin and yang within your creative process. Are you "yin dominant" or "yang dominant"? The more you understand how these forces show up in your work, relationships, and life, the more deeply you will understand the energies that make up your innate nature. You can then affirm what a natural flow feels like to you versus the feeling of excessive effort.

Rather than pushing, pulling, and exerting yourself, what if you were to get out of the way and listen to the stillness, feel, and see what is asking to be born? What if you were to take deep, spacious breaths and stop the "doing"? To pause and ask: Is this necessary, timely, and true—or is it just to keep busy? Listen to the whispers in the pause, in the stopping. Less is more. No pushing, no expectations, no judging. Only seeing with the eyes of a child: fresh, present, and willing to invite surprise and wonder.

As you listen deeply to each new experience without analyzing or thinking too much, you can feel into whether your yin or your yang energy best serves the moment. With practice, it will become easier to recognize when you are forcing and striving and when you are playing and being guided by intuition, curiosity, and a sense of being at one with the creative process. Sometimes you will still get caught in wanting things to be a certain way, but if you can recognize the feeling of allowing flow versus the feeling of controlling and forcing, you will know when you may be forcing the creative process and can pause to listen more deeply.

In this stillness, you can touch qualities of your core human nature that are waiting to be acknowledged and uncovered. You are a perfect, whole, and miraculous being, just as you are. There is no need to feel less than enough, to be fixed, or to fit into society's idea of who you should be. Circumstances are also perfect as they are—even if they are difficult, filled with impermanence, disappointing, or challenging. We are strengthening our ability to accept what *is*.

WEEK 5 INTENTIONS

During this week of the MBSE program, you will begin:

- To understand that light and dark are the yin and yang that make up all experience.

- To practice accepting yin and yang energies in your life, a balance that is always changing in an improvisational, natural rhythm moment to moment.

- To explore how you can choose to respond to any given circumstance with yin or yang energy, experimenting with different responses and experiencing things freshly, as if for the first time.

- To challenge fixed ideas and judgments, which are preconceived ideas, stories, beliefs and habits regarding what you consider to be good or bad, better or worse.

A new practice this week is the loving-kindness meditation, an open-hearted practice used to develop compassion, beginning with self-acceptance and then extending out to acceptance for others. This is how we heal rather than judge, criticize, and feel not good enough or separate and disconnected. This meditation embraces who we are, no matter what our circumstances, mistakes, and present conditions. It nurtures the awareness, understanding, acceptance, and wisdom to see things clearly and choose consciously how to respond, especially when experiencing darkness, illness, challenge, loss, or mistakes.

WEEK 5 DAILY PRACTICE

The list below details your practice for week 5. Read through it and, if you like, use it to prepare in advance for the week's practice. You can download a printable version of this list at https://www.newharbinger.com/44932 and post it in a place where you can see it easily. Visit the same URL to download the Art of Mindfulness Practice Guide, which contains directions for the body scan, sitting meditation, loving-kindness meditation, and gentle stretching yoga. (Audio guides for these practices are available there, too.)

1. Practice one of the week 5 Mindful Art Encounters (in the sections that follow) every day.

2. Alternate a body scan with gentle stretching yoga every other day.

3. Practice a sitting meditation each day for twenty minutes, paying attention to the breath and body sensations. (If twenty minutes is too long, try a five- or ten-minute version.) You may also want to incorporate the loving-kindness meditation into your sitting practice. A guide for loving-kindness meditation can be found in the downloadable Art of Mindfulness Practice Guide.

4. Explore options for responding mindfully and creatively and with a more spacious, open view. Use your breath as an anchor to the present moment, a means to increase awareness of reactive patterns. Bring awareness to your natural rhythm of breathing, following the inhalation and the exhalation, knowing when you are breathing in and when you are breathing out. After following for a few breaths, you can make more conscious choices.

5. Practice mindful awareness of feeling stuck, blocked, numb, or shut off to the moment whenever it happens this week.

6. Complete the Reflecting on the Week section at the end of this chapter.

Mindful Art Encounter #18: Exploring Yin and Yang

Materials: Two pieces of paper, colorful assortment of crayons and/or pencils, pen or pencil, journal

Do you have judgments against strong yang energy, leaning instead toward yin energy? Or perhaps you prefer yang energy? In this art encounter, we'll take a deeper look at your relationship to the yin and yang energies within and how you show up in the world.

Part 1: Yin

Yin energy is flow: open and accepting, receptive and fluid, like a river. Feel into your body and feel the rhythm of your breath as it flows in and out naturally. Begin to feel into colors that reflect the energy of yin: fluid, receptive, flexible, soft, and sensitive.

Create a composition with marks, shapes, lines, and colors that communicates your relationship to yin. For example, your lines might be curvy and round to reflect flow and fluidity. Or, your page might be made up of different-sized circles. Play with position and composition and use your imagination. How would you like to express being receptive and nurturing? What colors are you inspired to use? Some circles may be colored and some not. You might just draw outlines of circles and play with circular patterns as you engage with doodling and the feeling of receptivity. Play, be curious, and have fun. Feel into your body as you express yin energy.

Notice how yin is present in your life: in relationships, attitudes, decisions, and ways you are in the world.

Do yin characteristics feel familiar to you? Do you feel receptive, nurturing, and open? Are you able to extend the nurturing that you offer others to yourself? Do you take care of yourself? How? Name five ways that you take care of yourself.

_____

_____

_____

_____

How have your yin qualities enhanced your life, and how have they held you back? Name specific instances and examples.

_____

_____

_____

_____

_____

_____

Part 2: Yang

Now, change. Feel into the yang energy: active, assertive, agitated, dominant, and fiery. Close your eyes and feel the breath in your body, calling up the sensation of yang energy.

Create a composition with marks, shapes, lines, and colors that communicates your relationship to yang. For example, your colors might be vivid and saturated to reflect intensity and fire. Or you may once again choose to create a composition of circles. How can you express assertiveness, action, and strong energy within the creative play of circles?

When you're finished, ask yourself: Is yang energy more familiar for you? Can you recall examples and specific moments when you have been aware of a strong yang point of view, perhaps taking a stand, being assertive, or saying no? When you have taken care of yourself with clarity and a strong protective voice?

_____

_____

_____

_____

_____

How have your yang qualities enhanced your life, and how have they held you back? Name specific instances and examples.

_____

_____

_____

_____

_____

_____

Place your two drawings side by side on the floor.

What have you learned about yourself in the context of yin and yang? Which is your most dominant characteristic, and how does the opposite show up in your relationships with people and in situations and circumstances?

_____

_____

_____

_____

What did this encounter tell you about your preferences, what you resist, and what your struggle may be?

_____

_____

_____

_____

When dealing with stressful situations, are you more passive or more aggressive? How so? Do you retreat, or do you stand strong and communicate openly?

_____

_____

_____

Now that you are aware of these tendencies, are there ways to bring mindfulness and balance to enhance your well-being?

_____

_____

_____

How is your engagement with others and situations affected by your attitudes and perceptions of yin versus yang? How can you invite in qualities that may be out of the box, free of habits, and grounded in self-compassion? Explore these attitudes and perceptions.

_____

_____

_____

How can the process of yin and yang flowing together and enhancing each other in harmony and balance enable you to live fully and joyfully with acceptance and gratitude?

_____

_____

_____

Any time you repeat this exercise, journal about your experience.

Mindful Art Encounter #19: Exploring Judgment

Materials: Piece of white paper, plate or other round object for tracing, white crayon, light gray crayon, dark gray crayon, black crayon, pen or pencil, journal

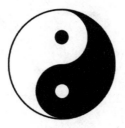

Look at the yin-yang symbol. What does it communicate to you? Do you know what it symbolizes in the world?

_____

_____

_____

_____

   This symbol represents how what seem to be opposing forces are actually complementary, interconnected, and interdependent. Light and dark, day and night—each can only exist with its opposite. The yin-yang symbolizes harmony between the two and the sacredness of wholeness.

   How can we celebrate both parts equally? Without one, we cannot have the other. Both are essential in the whole. We may have judgments, preferences, and unconscious biases about either side. Our judgments can influence how we feel about ourselves and others. Self-compassion leads to fewer judgments, kinder acceptance, and the realization of interconnectedness.

   Now close your eyes and take three deep breaths, coming into the present moment.

   Take the piece of paper and draw a circle in the center (or use a plate or other round object to trace one). Then, using your four crayons, take three minutes to make an abstract drawing of beliefs you have about yourself or others that are critical, diminishing, harsh, or unkind. Do not draw particular images or objects; rather, use shape, form, dark or light marks, angular or round lines, texture, and color.

   How can you express judgment that is unkind, that does not create joy for yourself or others? Focus on your personal experience and the feeling in your body when you call up positions that are unkind or repressive. There is no right or wrong way to express this feeling, no good or bad drawing. Create an image that expresses how judgment feels in your body. For example: you may feel sensations of contraction and tension.

When you are finished, close your eyes and feel the sensations in your body. Then, answer the following questions.

How are you feeling?

_____

_____

_____

Did this experience open your perception and understanding of how your body reacts to judging and being judged?

_____

_____

_____

Were you able to feel the connection between the judging thoughts, emotions, and sensations in your body? How did it feel? Where did you feel it in your body?

_____

_____

_____

Any time you repeat this exercise, journal about your experience.

Mindful Art Encounter #20: Exploring Acceptance

Materials: Drawing from Mindful Art Encounter #19, piece of white paper, plate or other round object to trace, white crayon, light gray crayon, dark gray crayon, black crayon, pen or pencil, journal

Close your eyes and take three deep breaths, coming into the present moment. Open your eyes and use a plate or other round object to trace a circle in the middle of your page. Then, use your four crayons to abstractly express feelings of joy, gratitude, open-heartedness, and kindness toward yourself and others. Fill the circle with expressions of acceptance and well-being. How can you express these feelings in line, shape, form, light, and dark? How do you feel as you draw a circular symbol of self-compassion, kindness, and open-heartedness? As you observe your drawing, does it communicate kindness to you? There is no right or wrong, no good or bad drawing. This encounter calls for you to feel kindness in your body and heart and express this feeling on paper.

When you have completed your drawing, close your eyes and feel into the sensations in your body. Then answer the following questions.

What are your emotions right now? How has this process been for you? Has it been possible to tap into and express the feeling of self-compassion?

_____

_____

_____

_____

How do these feelings show up in your body? For example, are you feeling relaxed, open, alive, expansive, playful, or free? Or guarded, closed, or having difficulty accessing a feeling of kindness?

_____

_____

_____

_____

How is this experience different from your experience in the previous encounter (#19) of exploring judgments? And how are the two experiences similar? What made them similar or different?

_____

_____

_____

_____

Notice how your body feels as you look at the drawing of joy and kindness. Be curious and see if there are any judgments about your drawing. Notice if when you are accepting of all experience without needing to judge, change, or evaluate a situation or another person, you can enter a space of expansive, kind acceptance, curiosity, and spaciousness. It is a generous opening to life as it flows in a natural rhythm rather than needing to control it through our personal preferences. Express in a few words how this process felt and where you felt it in your body.

_____

_____

_____

Retrieve your drawing from the previous art encounter and place it next to this one on the floor. Spend a few moments taking in the drawings: observing, looking, and seeing. Notice what happens in your belly when you observe the drawing of judgments. Is there a contraction, a feeling of resistance, a judgment of it being good or bad? Are you then judging that you're judging, adding another layer of judgment? Write your thoughts below, and then set your drawings aside.

_____

_____

_____

_____

Any time you repeat this exercise, journal about your experience.

Mindful Art Encounter #21: Embracing Yin and Yang

Materials: Drawings from Mindful Art Encounters #19 and #20, piece of white or black paper, plate or other round object for tracing, white crayon, light gray crayon, dark gray crayon, black crayon, pen or pencil, journal

Close your eyes and take three deep breaths, coming into the present moment. Be with whatever feelings you may be experiencing.

Our human experience includes both light and dark, judgment and kindness, criticism and light-heartedness. How can you create a drawing that uses mark-making to express both yin and yang?

Gather the four crayons and your white or black piece of paper. Use a plate or other round object to trace a circle in the middle of your paper. Then, awaken the opposing forces of yin and yang within you and express this relationship—this interaction—in your circle, using shape, tone, line, and dots.

Making marks is simple, and yet when we try to express the opposing forces that lie within and throughout nature and life, it can become a rich exploration informed by feelings, emotions, and expression of the opposites that dwell within. Lines can be light and dark, thick and thin, wide and narrow. Forms may be light, dark, overlapping, big, small, aggressive, joyful, contracted, or free. When you create a line inspired by anger and frustration, counter with another line that is joyful, peaceful, and inclusive. Think about music and how the notes denote emotions, feelings, sensations, and ideas; then do the same with marks. This can be frustrating before you get started. Do not give up. Once you have broken the ice, a whole new world of self-expression may open up, and you will be able to explore all human experience in this abstract way.

Rather than analyze, just begin and let things flow rather than trying to understand and adhere to instructions. There is no one way, so find *your* way to begin, even if you are not absolutely clear. Interpret the instructions and then let inspiration and improvisation take you on a journey. This journey may take you down a path that is a detour, and you may feel lost. Trust and see what happens. Remember that above all, you are learning to listen to your intuition, and this overrides any instruction. The only instruction is to be present. In the creative process, as in life, instruction is simply a jumping-off point. Then go where you are being led from within.

This exercise is an exploration of being creative when dark moments or difficult feelings arise. Also, what happens when you are happy? Can you accept happiness without downplaying it?

If you feel judgments arise, pause before reacting and explore what is happening inside you. Can there be a kind response? With whatever arises, pause, take a deep breath, and notice what is happening. Then act intentionally, rather than impulsively. Notice how it feels to engage without judging or reacting. How can you stay connected to your center, your source of creative expression?

Retrieve your drawings from art encounters #19 and #20 and place them beside this one on the floor. Each of these expressions is part of your being. Compare the drawings. Do you tend to default to yin or to yang?

We lean toward habitual, safe, familiar ways of being: yin fluidity or yang fixed. Sometimes a situation may call us to stretch beyond our habitual responding—beyond our narrow ego and a perspective that only considers our point of view—to pause and see a wider view. Look at the big picture with kindness, consideration, self-compassion, and compassion for all. By opening to a wider view, we may find a more powerful and intentional way of being. Which action serves the highest good in this moment? This practice introduces a whole new dimension of seeing the world and each other. It calls us to be awake, aware, and open-hearted as we recognize our place in the world and how our voice matters. Sometimes resistance is what is called for, and sometimes more open inclusivity and flow.

This may be challenging. You won't always get it right. It is important not to beat yourself up. You can learn from your mistakes. You are learning to be more aware. In this way, judging becomes an opportunity to practice what strengthens you and your connection to your innate creative source that, when accessed, flows through you and creates more joy.

Any time you do this exercise, journal about your experience.

REFLECTING ON THE WEEK

When you finish the week's work, take some time to reflect. Write in your journal or on the blank lines on whichever of the reflections or prompts below speak to you.

Reflections

- Yin and yang energies exist in all things. They may seem like opposites, but it is the flowing energy between them that creates the innate rhythms all around us and within us.

- The patterns of yin and yang within our bodies are deeply connected to the rhythms of the world around us, transforming and changing in each passing moment. Nothing stays the same.

- The balance of yin and yang is different for each of us. When you understand the dynamic tension between them that exists within you and creates your uniqueness, you can surrender to the natural flow that brings you alive.

Journal Prompts

Write down your own reflections of this week. What discoveries did you make? Any ahas?

_____

_____

_____

_____

_____

_____

How can you bring a friendlier, less judgmental attitude to yourself? What are three things you can do each day to care for yourself? For example, are there things that you find enjoyable and could do more regularly, such as going for a walk, taking a nap, soaking in the bath, listing to music, or speaking to a friend?

_____

_____

_____

_____

Give an example of a time when you have called on your strengths to overcome the notion of not feeling good enough.

_____

_____

_____

_____

How can you comfort, support, offer relief, console, and calm yourself in times of difficulty?

_____

_____

_____

_____

What brings you closer to joy? To feeling safe and protected? Closer to feeling love—not love from the outside, but that which comes from within?

_____

_____

_____

_____

After you have written, close your eyes and notice your emotions, your thoughts, and the sensations in your body.

Communicating

The true essence of humankind is kindness.

—Often attributed to the 14th Dalai Lama

Over the past five weeks, you have been examining past habits, patterns of emotional expression, and how you present yourself in everyday life. You are cultivating the capacity to be more flexible, more resilient, to recover more rapidly during challenging situations. This week you'll shift your focus to *interpersonal mindfulness*, an excellent space to practice staying aware and maintaining balance, especially under difficult conditions or in times of stress.

Relationships—with a spouse, children, a boss, coworkers, employees, friends, neighbors, even strangers—form a large part of our lives and can be an area of great stress. Challenges in relating might include brutality versus kindness, stinginess versus generosity, dismissal versus support, competitiveness versus alignment, divisiveness versus inclusivity, prejudice versus acceptance, and so on. The circle of relating can be one of great suffering but is also one in which the practices and insights that we've been learning in MBSE can be most helpful.

We are always interacting and communicating with others, and often our buttons are pushed in our closest relationships. We react automatically out of old habits, and before we know it, we are repeating the same interactions for the hundredth time. But what if we were able to experience this difficult communication as if for the very first time? What if, when we felt the familiar sensations of anger in our body—adrenaline rising up the spine, getting hot and sweaty, pulse quickening—we recognized that we had a choice? We can be reactive in the moment, having an outburst and intensifying the situation. Or we can pause, take three deep breaths, feel the sensations as they arise, and, with spaciousness and patience, diffuse the storm by letting go of fixed ideas and needing a particular outcome—usually to be right or to win. What if you let things be, invited acceptance and cooperation, and trusted the outcome?

Note that this choice can only exist in the presence of self-awareness, self-compassion and balance. We *must* be *aware* of what is happening in the moment: feelings, thoughts, sensations in our body, and how we are communicating to the other person. At the same time, we *must* maintain *balance* during a

Understanding the Eight Attitudes of Mindfulness

When practiced with kind attention and intention, these eight foundational attitudes cultivate a sense of well-being, right action, right speech, and right living, with less striving, less needing things to be different, and less expectations of self and others. It is a wholesome and beautiful way to live kindly, peacefully, and in harmony.

1. *Beginners' mind* is a willingness to see things as if for the very first time, with curiosity and a sense of wonder. No matter what the experience or with whom—tasting a mango, being with a friend, feeling the wind on your skin, the warm embrace of a partner—beginner's mind allows us to be open to a new experience each time, aware and awake to the present moment. One of my favorite examples of this is the raisin exercise in week 2. How would you experience a raisin for the very first time? Beginner's mind enables us to experience each precious moment in our lives, rather than missing the moments in a blur of busy-ness, judgment, and expectations. A participant in the program broke down as she looked at photos of family vacations in exquisite locations, realizing that she could not remember anything about the experiences. Where was she? What had she been so preoccupied with? Her expensive holidays had come and gone, and the only thing she had was the photographs. She had not been present in her life.

2. *Nonjudgment* means moving beyond preferences, opinions, likes and dislikes, and good and bad to be a neutral observer of our experience. So much energy is exerted in preferences of liking and disliking, pushing away what we do not like and pulling toward us what we like and often want more of. Nonjudgment is a release of this energy, witnessing what we are experiencing without judging or reacting.

stormy interaction or repetitive stressful encounter, like a mountain that remains unchanged no matter what the weather or how frequently it storms.

In her inspiring book *The Four-Fold Way*, Angeles Arrien discusses four attitudinal qualities of mindfulness and how they can transform our relationships by changing the way we communicate. The four qualities she outlines are:

1. choosing to be generously open and present without judgments

2. heartfelt witnessing and listening to what is being expressed by the other

3. speaking without preferences, blame, or judgments, rooted in the present moment

4. allowing what is without trying to influence the outcome, fix, or change anything.

3. *Acceptance* is being with things as they are in the present moment, without needing to change them in any way—even when they are not as we would prefer. There is no need to be invested or disinvested; just be neutral and accepting. Open your palms to receive, letting go of personal preferences.

4. *Patience* enables us to allow things to unfold in their own time. There is an innate wisdom and time for everything. Rather than anticipating and expecting, soften to what *is* and accept that it will change in a rhythm that is beyond your expectations and anticipations.

5. *Trust*, or self-reliance, allows us to listen deeply to our own inner wisdom and innate experience. We trust the flow of things as they are and that everything fits together into one whole, living, breathing world. Self-reliance and self-compassion are beautiful, affirming ways to acknowledge that we trust the process and are able to take care of ourselves with kind attention.

6. *Non-striving* is about allowing things to unfold in a natural way, without pushing, striving, or expending too much effort. Loosen the grip, being aware of things without needing to control them or specify an outcome.

7. *Letting be* means releasing ourselves from preferences, opinions, and wanting things to be different, swimming with the current rather than against the tide. Sometimes we need to just float and trust, surrendering to the larger energy that is all around and within.

8. *Kindness* enables us to be generous in giving and receiving, listening and speaking, and being present with empathy. Kindness also means feeling gratitude for things as they are.

Arriens's four qualities are inspired by the eight attitudes of mind that form the core of mindfulness and which we have already been practicing throughout our journey: beginner's mind, nonjudgment, acceptance, patience, trust (self-reliance), non-striving, letting be, and kindness to self and others. Each of these attitudes relies on all the others; they are interconnected. When you work on one, you are working on all of them.

The practice of mindfulness is similar to planting a garden. There are certain conditions necessary for a garden to flourish and bloom: plenty of sunshine, enough water, and rich soil. In the same way, the eight attitudes of mindfulness are necessary for our lives to flourish. When we cultivate these attitudes with attention, intention, and practice, we are nourishing, strengthening, and supporting the garden of our life by committing to be awake and aware as each precious moment unfolds. As we do so, these attitudes naturally spill over into our relations with others. Here are some examples of how the eight attitudes of mindfulness can guide our communication with others:

- Opening a space for kind consideration by seeing the other as ourselves.

- Putting ourselves in the other person's shoes, understanding that we are all in this process of life together.

- Choosing to be okay with not having to be right or get our own way, and not seeing the situation from only one point of view.

- Meeting the other person and ourselves as one, understanding that we are all interconnected.

- Understanding that every action causes waves of either kindness (increasing love and understanding) or cruelty (selfishness that causes harm and disconnect).

- Knowing that meanness, callousness, cruelty, bullying, striving, and competition all fuel separation, as opposed to harmony, flow, and kind collaboration.

- Seeing all experience as interconnected coexistence, calling for right action, right speech, right livelihood, and right relationships based on trust and kindness.

These attitudes are simple and yet difficult to practice in real life. When I teach the MBSE workshops to law students, for example, most of the students begin the workshop with some skepticism. They make fun of meditation and the creative process. They become impatient when we begin the body scan, wiggling and whispering to their neighbors. Some even ask to leave the room. As they resist, I feel my own judgment and impatience begin to build. I have to remind myself that this is a habitual pattern. I remind myself to not hold fast to outcomes, instead opening the space for anything to happen. No goals in mind, no expectations, no striving—just an open heart and trust that I am coming from an authentic place as I share my experience of this process and how it saved my life.

We usually want to dive in, react, and give opinions. We close the spacious circle of acceptance because it may feel uncomfortable, preferring to fill it with words, ideas, recommendations, opinions, and our points of view. The next time you are communicating with someone, try to be as quiet as possible. Let them speak, and open spaces for pauses and stillness without jumping in to fill them. This is an act of generosity, trust, and gratitude for the other person's sharing. Let go of your habitual ways of responding and reacting and instead trust the process of silence, simplicity, and letting things be. Remain open, non-judgmental, patient, present with beginner's mind, trusting, and non-striving. Accept things as they are, letting go of outcome.

If and when you do speak, take a deep breath first and exhale into the moment. Pause. Become aware of your intention. Think about what you are about to say and ask yourself:

- Is it kind?

- Is it true?

- Is it necessary?

- Is it timely?

- Is it judgmental?

- Is it intended to enhance the relationship?

- Is it controlling?

- Is it a tool to justify my position or elevate myself in the eyes of the other person?

- Is it biased?

- Is it my interpretation?

- Is it intended to bring me closer to one person at the expense of another?

- Is it to gain attention, position, confidence, or approval?

- Is it to make me feel superior?

Kind Speech Is *Not*:

- Accusations

- Idle gossip

- Manipulation

- Revenge

- Meant to establish superiority or intellect

Kind Speech *Is*:

- Uniting

- Loving

- Empathetic

- Compassionate

- Considerate

- Patient

- Soft

- Expansive of heart and being

- Nourishing to self and others

Are your words cultivating a rich and flourishing interaction, or are they planting seeds of hate and discontent? Engaging in gossip is the same no matter whether you are the speaker or listener. If you're involved in a stressful communication, one approach is to use the following construct:

When you [name a specific behavior], I felt [name a specific emotion] because [name the reason it made you feel that way]. In the future, can you please [request a specific change in behavior]?

Think back on a recent challenging encounter in your life. How did it feel in your body? Ill will creates negativity and discomfort for ourselves, even if it was intended for another. Being unkind affects us directly and is detrimental to our well-being and sense of ease.

- How do you feel after speaking with intention?

_____

- How do you feel after speaking unkindly?

_____

- How do you feel after speaking with anger?

_____

- How do you feel after speaking from a desire to control, manipulate, or demean?

_____

The way we communicate with others is a direct reflection of our own inner dialogue. In other words, you cannot give what you do not have. Nurture self-compassion and the space of generosity within yourself so sharing is simply part of the flow of love and kind connection. This way, when a blow comes your way, you have the inner resources and strength to choose how to respond. This may sound impossible. We are human, after all. Habits are deeply ingrained and have taken years to form. We make mistakes, and we screw up. This is why it is called *practice*. We can practice over and over and over again.

Let's acknowledge that you are doing your best. Becoming aware of your habits is being mindful, and once you have awareness, you can choose how to act. Of course, being familiar with your habits does not mean that you'll no longer react in the moment. But our practice is about bringing kind compassion to each moment, even when we are *un*mindful. Always come back to the present moment with acceptance and nonjudgment. Every moment is a chance to begin again.

As you've been learning, the experience of living is abundant with difficulties and joys—yin and yang. Light requires darkness to shine, and darkness requires light—there are great gifts in both. The same holds true for relationships. Even challenging relationships offer great gifts: opportunities to strengthen your voice and practice being assertive rather than passive, aggressive, or passive-aggressive. State your needs clearly so as to be heard and to discern what feels right versus unhealthy. From this new strength, you can choose how to take care of yourself and what to engage with or disconnect from as you listen to the voice inside.

WEEK 6 INTENTIONS

During this week of the MBSE program, you will begin:

- To understand that you have a choice in how you communicate with others.

- To become aware that nurturing your inner dialogue through the eight attitudes of mindfulness is the most important way to foster self-compassion and less stressful relations with others.

- To practice kind speech in all communications, including challenging ones.

WEEK 6 DAILY PRACTICE

The list below details your practice for week 6. Read through it and, if you like, use it to prepare in advance for the week's practice. You can download a printable version of this list at http://www.newhar binger.com/44932 and post it in a place where you can see it easily. Visit the same URL to download the Art of Mindfulness Practice Guide, which contains directions for the body scan, sitting meditation, loving-kindness meditation, and gentle stretching yoga. Audio guides for these practices are available there, too, as is a printable file of the Difficult Communications Calendar (this can also be found at the back of this book).

1. Do one of the week 6 Mindful Art Encounters (in the sections that follow) every day.

2. Each day, alternate a body scan with gentle stretching yoga.

3. Do a sitting meditation for five minutes each day, paying attention to your breath and body sensations.

4. Commit to practicing kind speech and the eight attitudes of mindfulness and notice how your life unfolds. Journal about your observations.

5. If you experience a challenging interaction with someone this week, fill out the Difficult Communications Calendar.

6. Each day, perform an act of generosity toward yourself and then to another. See how this feels. As you go through your day, recognize moments of gratitude.

7. Complete the Reflecting on the Week section at the end of this chapter.

Mindful Art Encounter #22: Listening Enemy or Friend?

Materials: Paper; art materials of your choosing, such as crayons, markers, black ink, pencils, glue, eraser, white correction fluid, found objects from nature; pen or pencil; journal

Note: Before starting this exercise, review the choiceless awareness section in the sitting meditation guide in the downloadable Art of Mindfulness Practice Guide found at http://www.newharbinger.com/44932.

Another important tool in our journey is choiceless awareness meditation, designed to bring greater awareness to whatever is happening in the present moment, whether a body sensation, a sound entering your ear, the feel of a breeze on your skin, a thought, pain or discomfort, and so on. We can only have one thought or experience in each moment, and each of us experiences an ever-changing, colorful kaleidoscopic of senses—tasting, seeing, touching, hearing, and smelling the richness of the world—in our own unique way. If we are lost in the past or the future, we are missing the whole experience of being present.

Start this art encounter by doing a sitting meditation for five minutes, following the downloadable audio or printable guide. As you do, focus your attention on any reactions, harsh judgments, criticisms, bullying, or aggression toward yourself. For example:

Why was I so stupid to think that?

What is this pain that is making me so crazy? I wish it would go away.

Why me?

Why can't I have what I want? I deserve it.

Why am I so fat?

I shouldn't be so sad. I'm being such a baby.

I don't like this practice. It's boring and a waste of time.

Notice how this type of inner dialogue feels as you process it in your body.

As your meditation comes to an end, gather the paper and art materials and recall a challenging encounter. Write your answers to the following questions:

• What happened?

• What were your thoughts?

- What were your feelings?

- What were your body sensations?

- What were your emotions?

- How did you react or respond?

_____

_____

_____

_____

_____

_____

_____

_____

_____

_____

On a piece of paper, draw and express the inner experience of challenge, contraction, judgment, opinions, aggression, bullying, and self-criticism as well as the reflection of this inner dialogue in the outer scenario of reactivity and hostility. When you are finished, set this drawing aside.

Now, think back on the same encounter, but this time, use the eight attitudinal qualities of mindfulness to imagine how it might have gone differently. Once again, write your answers to the following:

- What happened?

- What were your thoughts?

- What were your feelings?

- What were your body sensations?

- What were your emotions?

- How did you react or respond?

_____

_____

_____

_____

_____

_____

_____

_____

_____

On a second piece of paper, express the new experience. What changed to make the second experience different? Were you able to practice the eight attitudes of mindfulness, and if so, what was the effect?

Remember, you can choose how you respond to situations—especially difficult ones. By introducing the eight attitudes of mindfulness, you may change the landscape of your life and your connection with others.

Any time you do this exercise, journal about your experience.

Mindful Art Encounter #23: Drawing and Collaging with Words

Materials: Pencils, crayons, markers, eraser, ten sheets of paper, glue stick or glue, scissors, magazines and newspapers you can cut up, stamps with words, letter stencils, pen or pencil, journal

Over the past weeks, you've become more familiar with automatic drawing, patterning, and discovery through the process of mark-making. Let's add to these processes by using collage. The goal of this encounter is to quickly do ten separate collages—one per minute. This is a playful way to practice letting go and being spontaneous, opening the door to surprise and new discoveries.

First, page through old magazines and newspapers and cut out words that attract you by their shape or meaning. You can also form your own words by cutting out letters of varied typefaces and placing them together.

When you have at least ten words, glue one of the words onto a piece of paper, and then spend one minute quickly drawing other words, phrases, shapes, designs, lines, and notes to yourself on and around the word to express what it inspires in your life. For example, if your word is "ballet," what does ballet mean in your life? Maybe it's a reminder of how much you miss dancing and feeling rhythm in your body. Even a word that seemed random when you selected it carries a message. Explore why it was chosen. Use your collage to communicate a message to yourself, perhaps something only you will understand and do not want to forget or a reminder to always take care of yourself and not expect someone else to fill the emptiness.

You might place your word in the middle of the page with lines extending outward. Or, place your word anywhere on the page and use it as a starting point for drawn lines, shapes, and dots. Remember, there is no wrong way. There are no mistakes. Quickly build a collage of inspirations, longings, reminders, messages, gratitude, and creative expressions.

As you add lines, shapes, notes, and dots, you can also subtract them with your eraser. This sometimes leaves a whisper of a mark, adding richness to the composition. Bold lines and cut-out words also make for a varied composition. The collage becomes a record of your experience, made mark by mark in the moment.

Allow the process to take you on a journey on the artful path of discovery. Risk making a mess or an ugly collage. Play and enjoy the process. Be bold. If you're going to make a mess, make a big one! Befriend fear. Befriend not feeling good enough. Befriend anxiety and not knowing what to do, not feeling creative, feeling stuck. Try new things. Let one moment lead to the next, making discoveries along the way. You are engaging in the process of change, moment to moment. You are engaging in the process of making choices, moment to moment. This is practice to strengthen, listen to, and trust spontaneity, your inner senses of direction and adventure.

As soon as you "finish" one collage, take another word and start the next one, quickly doing all ten in ten minutes.

If you feel like you've messed up, check in with yourself. How are you? What is your inner dialogue, and how do you carry on to the next mark or word? Bring kind expression and generous listening to the process. As each collage evolves, pause, stop, and listen to what is needed rather than just carrying on to the next word or mark.

Experiential drawing and collage are windows to seeing into your life in a new way. Are you finding this experience surprising and inspiring? Or are you stressed, trying too hard, exerting too much effort? The collages illuminate how you speak to yourself, which in turn reflects how you communicate with others. Is your process full of harsh words and criticism? Or inspiring, kind, empowering words?

Words can hurt, and words can enhance and inspire. Often, we speak without thinking, but right speech calls for pause, awareness, and intention. The inner work of mindfulness leads to a kinder inner dialogue of self-compassion, which in turn leads to more compassionate outer communication. The two are reflections of each other. We can begin again in this moment and change how we speak, adding kindness and generous support. Treat the collages as vision boards to bring the eight attitudinal qualities of mindfulness into your life.

When you have finished all ten collages, stop. Breathe into the moment, take a long pause, and observe. Your handwriting is your visual voice. Look at the gestures, marks, and spaces in between and answer these questions.

What is your emotional state right now? Where are you feeling tension in your body?

_____

_____

_____

What are your thoughts?

_____

_____

_____

_____

What did you learn from this encounter that you may not have been aware of before?

_____

_____

_____

_____

What thinking patterns were you aware of while cutting, tearing, and pasting? What was surprising?

_____

_____

_____

_____

How did it feel as you patched things together with your personal notes, lines, and patterns? Have you chartered any new territory?

_____

_____

_____

_____

Any time you repeat this exercise, journal about your experience.

Mindful Art Encounter #24: Engaged Listening

Materials: Watercolor paper; black ink; thin, medium, and thick paintbrushes; a device to play music and music of your choosing; pen or pencil; journal

Two of the most important aspects of mindfulness are practicing silence and spaciousness. Rather than filling each moment with activity, distractions, words, doing, or planning, you are learning to open up spaces of non-doing and emptiness. It is within these empty spaces that inspiration may arise. In listening to your intuition and inner guidance, you may replenish, heal, and feel at ease.

Play music of your choosing; let it enter your body. Feel the rhythm, energy, and emotions inspired by the notes. Take three deep breaths. Dip your brush in ink and pause. When you feel inspired, make your first mark. Pause and take three more deep breaths. Load the brush again and wait until the moment when you are inspired to make another mark. Continue listening to the music, making marks in response to the sound.

When you feel you have made your marks, place the brush down and take some time to just look at them. Take them in visually as well as through sensations in your body and emotions. Connect with the marks as experience rather than *thinking* about the marks. If you begin to judge the marks, label the judgments and then come back to the experience of the marks on the paper. Try to leave thinking out of the experience. If it happens, notice that thinking has occurred and then return to the experience. The marks are a creative expression of your experience.

What are the sensations in your body? Are you feeling free, released, inspired, wanting to do more? Or are you feeling restricted and contracted?

Now, think about your relationship to listening—not only to sounds, but to the space between the sounds.

Play the music again.

Do you feel the pauses, the silence between the sounds, and what they add to the musical experience?

_____

_____

Do you feel comfortable in silent moments? Or are you uncomfortable?

_____

_____

What is the soundtrack for your life? What are the words, and how do they communicate?

_____

_____

_____

_____

_____

Do you often have sound on in your life, such as from TV, music, radio, podcasts, or background chatter?

_____

Can you be alone in silence? How do you relate when silence is there?

_____

_____

_____

How can you take this lesson into your life? Give an example.

_____

_____

_____

_____

Any time you repeat this exercise, journal about your experience.

Mindful Art Encounter #25: Listening to Your Whispers

Materials: Paper, art materials of your choosing, pen or pencil, journal

As you invite silence, simplicity, and solitude into your life, you may notice that you begin to feel into what your inner whispers are saying. This spacious listening may feel uncomfortable at first. Be patient. Don't become discouraged. In time, it may lead you to insights about what is important to you, what you cannot live without, and what inspires and ignites joy.

This is a powerful practice and a gift. It is in this quiet space, away from distraction and noise, that you may almost hear your heart beating, feel your pulse rhythmically pushing blood though your veins, feel the weather of your emotions and body sensations. You may notice that you begin to feel into the rhythm of your breathing. Is your breathing shallow or deep, long or short? Where do you feel it most vividly in your body? As you connect to the breathing, you also connect to the present moment.

Create a quiet place for yourself and spend a few minutes simply sitting in the silence. Then, answer the following questions.

What fascinates you and enriches your life? What do you care about?

_____

_____

_____

_____

Do you enjoy being busy, rushing, and feeling adrenalin? Do you like to be scheduled from one moment to the next without spaces in between to do nothing and simply be?

_____

_____

Do you prefer being with others or by yourself? Do you like to talk or prefer to be quiet?

_____

_____

Do you enjoy being out in nature, on the ocean, or in the forest?

_____

_____

Does silence feed you and fill you up or make you feel uncomfortable?

_____

_____

We are all sailing the boat of our life. How do you wish to move through the water? Take three deep breaths and then use your art materials to draw your boat on the water. Place it anywhere on the paper. Your boat can be as simple as a circle or a dot.

What would you like to have with you in your boat of life? These do not have to be big things; they can be tiny meaningful experiences. Who would you like to invite aboard? Use words, signs, shapes, lines, and marks to denote all the people and things you would like in your boat. Then, ask yourself: What do I want to leave behind? Maybe see those things floating nearby or in a pile on shore. For example, how much technology do you want in the boat? Is it enhancing or detracting from your engagement with life?

Using your imagination, be playful and have fun. Play with the visuals. Erase and experiment, rather than trying to make a perfect drawing. Think of this as a quirky illustration. Allow it to be messy, ugly, not serious or perfect.

As you focus inward, bring awareness to what is enhancing your life. What is holding you back? Try not to criticize, judge, and hold fixed views. Kindness, radical acceptance, self-compassion, and love of life open space for new experiences to enter. This is a powerful opportunity to listen deeply and assess your life from the inside rather than have it be dictated by outer forces. This is not easy. We are so used to being outer-focused.

When you are finished, pause, then answer the following questions:

Has this experience helped you shed light on what you would like to include in your life and what to let go of? What do you really need? What are your core values? How can you take care of yourself?

_____

_____

_____

What are you tolerating in your life right now?

_____

_____

_____

_____

What do you need to invite more of?

_____

_____

_____

_____

Do you have kind, supportive friends and community?

_____

_____

_____

How are the drawing encounters informing your experiences? Does the visual language of drawing allow you to see things differently, or not? Does it compliment the formal and informal mindfulness exercises?

_____

_____

_____

Any time you repeat this exercise, journal about your experience.

Mindful Art Encounter #26: Conversation Drawing with a Partner

Materials: Two pieces of paper, art materials of your choice, pen or pencil, journal

So far the MBSE journey has been a journey of going inward and shining a light on deeper understanding with kind acceptance and self-compassion. Now, almost like a coming-out party, you will invite another to join you in the conversation.

Part 1

Begin by facing another person with a piece of drawing paper between you. Take a moment to breathe and become present. Without speaking, take turns having a visual conversation with your partner in the form of marks, shapes, lines, colors, and textures on the paper. Notice what is happening inside of you, paying attention to the feelings and sensations in your body.

When it is your turn, is there excitement, apprehension, tension? If a judging or critical voice arises, just notice it. Check in with your breath: Is it moving freely, or is there constriction? This exercise is an opportunity to cultivate kindness through responding creatively to your partner as well as yourself.

Stay present and notice your partner's mark, listening attentively to its expression. Is it gentle, energetic, or colorful? Playful or serious? Notice your perception of his or her mark and respond creatively. Is it easier to listen or to express yourself?

Explore and play. See what you discover. What color is exciting? What shapes are you interested in? Are you playing it safe or taking risks? Does the conversation feel like a flow of exchange, each partner enhancing what is being expressed? How does it feel to be in the present moment of mark-making with no idea what the final drawing will look like? How does it feel to not have control or work toward a specific goal? Are you able to trust what is being revealed moment to moment? Are you able to let go when your partner makes marks that you do not care for? Can you open a space for acceptance and allowing, even when you do not like what he or she has done?

Part 2

Working together, rip up the drawing. Tear it into as many pieces as you wish.

Notice how you feel as you rip up the drawing. Is there resistance? Sadness? Anger? A feeling of loss and wanting to save this thing that the two of you have created? Or is there a sense of surprise, surrender, and an opening to new possibility? There may be a feeling of wild abandon and excitement, of letting go into spontaneous possibility. How do you feel as you continue ripping and as the drawing becomes less and less recognizable?

When you've finish ripping, put the pieces down. Take three deep breaths. Close your eyes and feel what is to be felt in the body. What thoughts, feelings, and sensations are you experiencing now? Allow the experience to be exactly as it is.

Open your eyes, slowly looking at the torn pieces. Do you see anything new?

Part 3

Together, move the pieces around on a fresh piece of paper and play with their relationships to one another. How many ways can you move them around? Try placing them overlapping, close to each other, far apart, joined, grouped, parallel, angled, diagonal, vertical, horizontal, with some folded to create three-dimensional forms, falling off the page, simplified, with space in between.

Notice the shapes of the spaces between the torn shapes. This is a new perspective. We are usually object-focused and do not see the spaces around the objects, which is often more interesting than the objects themselves. Can you let go of your attachment to the objects and open your perspective to seeing spaces that the objects inhabit? Experiment. Begin to see how, moment to moment, slow looking and seeing freshly can form new perspectives and a new composition that may not have been revealed before.

Explore relationships as you glue the pieces down. Are there any surprises or fresh inspirations? Slowly let go of the old creation as it begins to fade into the past and a new composition emerges.

Any time you do this exercise, journal about your experience.

REFLECTING ON THE WEEK

When you finish the week's work, take some time to reflect before going on. Write in your journal or on the blank lines on whichever of the reflections or prompts below speak to you.

Reflections

- Relationships can be a source of stress but are also an area where the practices and skills gained through MBSE can be of most use.

- Mindful communication requires awareness (of emotions, sensations, and thoughts experienced in the moment) and balance.

- Rather than react to outer hostility and anger, you can pause and choose how to respond, diffusing the storm through kind speech and the eight attitudes of mindfulness.

- The way you communicate with others is a reflection of your own inner dialogue: inner and outer are reflections of each other. The most important work you can do is to nurture compassion, self-love, and kindness.

Journal Prompts

Write down your reflections of this week. What discoveries did you make? Any ahas?

_____

_____

_____

_____

_____

_____

What did you discover about your emotions and sensations this week? How do your thoughts impact your words? How are thoughts, emotions, and sensations connected?

_____

_____

_____

_____

_____

Where do you feel aggression and anger in your body during stressful communication? How do they manifest as sensations (for example, sweaty palms, contracted belly, racing heart, headache, feeling flushed and hot)?

_____

_____

_____

_____

_____

When you feel connected and warm in communication, what do you feel (for example, relaxed, connected and aligned, safe, a feeling that "all is right with the world," trusting, whole, a sense of belonging to the world)?

_____

_____

_____

_____

Review the eight attitudinal qualities of mindfulness and give specific examples of how you incorporated them into your communications this week. How did they change each interaction?

_____

_____

_____

_____

_____

_____

_____

_____

A Retreat of Silence, Simplicity, and Solitude

When we can be centered in ourselves, even for brief periods of time in the face of the pull of the outer world, not having to look elsewhere for something to fill us up or make us happy, we can be at home wherever we find ourselves, at peace with things as they are, moment by moment.

—Jon Kabat-Zinn, *Wherever You Go, There You Are*

This week we're going to do something a little different, creating a space to pause and reflect. There are no new mindful art encounters. Instead, we'll continue with our daily practice and, most importantly, schedule a personal retreat day. This retreat day is for you to marinate and enjoy "not doing." It is a day to immerse yourself in practice and repeat any mindful art encounters that feel right for you. No distractions. No technology. It is a day all to yourself—to nourish yourself, play, and enjoy the space of befriending your experience as it is.

Throughout the week, continue to practice forty minutes each day of sitting meditation, gentle stretching yoga, walking meditation, or body scan meditation. If you cannot do the full forty minutes, create a practice that works for you. Remember, the important thing is to practice and to be kind to yourself. Feel free to blend practices, such as ten minutes of yoga followed by twenty-five minutes of sitting practice. Or, start with an awareness of breath meditation for twenty minutes and then add a ten- to fifteen-minute body scan or loving-kindness meditation. Experiment and create a practice that resonates. Planning and scheduling a time are important so you know that this is your time for your regular daily practice. Try going without recordings or using a recording every second day, whatever feels easier.

If you cannot set aside a full day for your retreat, decide how much time you can spend for yourself, even if only a couple hours. Stretch this a little beyond what you feel you can do. Get out of your comfort zone, even if it feels impossible. More time will allow you to deepen your practice. Remember, when you have an appointment with a doctor or business associate, you stay for as long as it takes because it is important to you. Treat yourself with the same importance and see what happens when you commit.

To get the most out of your retreat day, find a quiet place where you will not be disturbed and gather the following:

- this book

- yoga mat

- chair or cushion (zafu)

- blanket

- warm layers of clothing

- art supplies and paper

- your journal

- water, lunch, and snacks

- book of your favorite poetry (optional)

- something to play the recordings on (if you'd like to listen any of the recordings that go with this book).

Being with yourself is enlightening but can also be shocking. When we're alone, we face life full-on. We're used to noise, busyness, and the distractions of daily life, which numb our heart and sense of inter-connectedness. Silence can offer a respite. It's in aloneness that our emotions, sensations, and thoughts can truly arise and offer us the opportunity to see clearly. As we speak less, we listen more. We become aware of our stories, assumptions, conclusions, judgments, concepts, and opinions and of how much of our reality is stuck in this place.

As you begin your retreat, I invite you to embrace the silence, the not knowing, and the unexplainable. Dive beneath the waves of restlessness and discover the stillness in silence. Listen deeply to the rhythms of your breath and your heart. As you enter each moment, listen deeply. The intimacy of silence can communicate many things, including:

- your deepest values and intention

- inspirations

- a clarity that may have not been there before

- renewal and healing

- creativity and strength

- deep sensitivity and harmony

- new possibilities and beginnings

- trust

- kindness

- rest

- stillness

- and the opposites as well.

Your retreat can unfold however you choose, as long as you commit to immersing yourself in practice imbued with kindness. If you prefer more structure, the schedule below offers one possible approach. Adjust it to work with whatever amount of time you have allowed.

9:00 a.m.	Start by asking yourself, "What is my intention for this precious time that I have gifted myself?" Write your answer below. _____ _____ _____
9:15 a.m.	15-minute body scan
9:30 a.m.	15-minute sitting meditation with attention on the breath
9:45 a.m.	15 minutes of gentle stretching yoga
10:00–11:30 a.m.	Redo the following mindful art encounters, taking however long you need • Mindful Art Encounter #1: Who Am I? • Mindful Art Encounter #6: Conversation Drawing with Self. Practice moment-to-moment attention, listening to your intuition, and being in the process rather than following goals and plans. • Mindful Art Encounter #7: Letting Go. Practice letting be and engaging with risk, doubt, vulnerability, and the spaciousness of not knowing. • Mindful Art Encounter #8: Rebuilding, Part 1. Surrender is the heart of letting go. Practice taking destroyed pieces and using them to create a new composition. • Mindful Art Encounter #9: Opening Your Reality. Practice seeing more clearly and opening up to a new reality of acceptance.
11:30 a.m.	Spend 15 minutes journaling. Ask yourself: • What has changed since I began this journey? • What are the practices teaching me? • Can I differentiate between thoughts, emotions, and sensations? Can I accept difficult emotions and sensations and know they are workable? • When I am stuck in thought, am I able to recognize that thoughts come and go and that I am not my thoughts? Write in stream-of-conscience style. Do not try to be clever or think too much. Keep your pen moving on the page without stopping. When you can't think of what to write, just write, "I can't think of what to write," and keep writing it until the time ends. When you're finished, put your pen or pencil down and close your eyes. Take three deep breaths. Feel into your body. What body sensations, thoughts, and feelings are you aware of in this moment?

11:45 a.m.	15-minute walking meditation (preferably outside, or inside if necessary)
Noon	Eat lunch, practicing mindful eating for 30 minutes.
12:30 p.m.	If you'd like, read from your book of poetry (if you brought one).
12:45 p.m.	5- or 8-minute sitting meditation
1:00 p.m.	Read more poetry of your choice and then take 5 minutes to journal about your inspirations and thoughts.
1:15 p.m.	Write a letter to yourself about things that have inspired you and that you do not want to forget. What do you want to do with this one wild and precious life?
1:30 p.m.	5- to 8-minute sitting meditation
1:45 p.m.	Spend 15 minutes journaling about your retreat, answering the following questions: • What was your experience of the time devoted to inner reflection? • What was your experience of the formal practices and mindful art encounters today? What was difficult, and what flowed? Any aha moments? • Were you able to find ways in which you engaged differently and where your dialogue was surprising and new? • How were you able to relate to difficulty differently? Were there gifts of recognition in the process? How can creative art encounters help you do this? Sometimes it is just plain hard, and there are no gifts that you can see. Give yourself a word of encouragement for staying with the process. When we struggle, we may learn that we can see things differently, in a far less attached way, and can choose a wider perspective. We can bring a lighter touch to experience.
2:00 p.m.	Make a list of five things that you are grateful for.
2:15 p.m.	End. Acknowledge yourself for taking the time to nourish yourself with silence, self-care, and peace.

Week 8

Going Deeper and Wider

No man is an island, entire of itself; every man is a piece of the continent, a part of the main…

—John Donne, *Devotions Upon Emergent Occasions*

The human condition is something we all experience and share in different ways. This week, you'll begin to explore how you relate with others and the world as a breathing, living whole. Walls that previously separated us may begin to dissolve as you tap into the innate creative goodness that we share. The interconnectedness of our humanity may feel like a big embrace as we begin to see a wider view of the vast blue sky above the clouds: spacious, open, and full of possibility.

We live in a patriarchal society of competition, winners, and losers. Many of us are ruled by fear, just trying to fit in. We contort and mask our true nature, attached to the impressions that we hope to communicate in an effort to be accepted. Rather than leading to acceptance and happiness, this exhausting process negates our true nature, our vulnerability, and our personal experiences, separating and disconnecting us from ourselves and each other. *An Artful Path to Mindfulness* is the personal journey of creating a meaningful life from the ground of genuine experience and self compassion. This is the art of living.

We *all* experience loss, challenges, disappointments, rejection, and failures. We *all* feel sadness, fear, anxiety, and jealousy, albeit in a unique way. Challenges and surprises are a part of living—for everyone. There is no controlling life.

It's by deepening your friendship with yourself—accepting who you are in all of your colors and shades of light and dark changing in each moment—that you are able to reach out to others in a similarly loving, genuine way. By loosening the grip of ego, letting go of empty self-promotion and the need for external approval, and relaxing into life unfolding, you may begin to experience your heart opening to self-acceptance, kindness, and sharing your experience without shame or judgment.

As you live your genuine experience, learn from others, and open yourself to vulnerability, the walls that separate us begin to dissolve, and we can relate to each other and the world as an interconnected, living, breathing whole. When we connect with others through our shared experience, we expand the footprint of our lives, deepening the richness and meaning of experience.

Begin Every Day Mindfully

When you wake up in the morning, instead of jumping out of bed and into the next thing, checking your phone or rushing and planning and preempting your day, lie quietly in bed for a few moments. Feel the sheets touching your skin, feel the bed supporting you, and feel the warmth that has been generated by your body.

As you lie still, what sensations are you feeling? Tired or energized? Is there any pain or discomfort? Do a short body scan: toes, feet, lower legs, upper legs, pelvis, buttocks, waist, stomach, upper body, shoulders, upper arms, lower arms, fingers, neck, head, face, crown. Feel into your body lying and being supported by the bed.

Acknowledge a sense of gratitude for this body that is so miraculous. No matter what ailments you may experience, there is more right than wrong with you.

Bring to mind five things that you are grateful for. Feel the sensation of gratitude in your body. How does it feel?

Set your intention for the day: to bring presence and kind attention to each moment, to be open and receptive, to be kind, to listen deeply and spaciously to whomever is speaking without opinions or the need to fix anything.

How much of life have you cut off through numbing and denial? The body has a language that speaks loudly and sometimes screams for us to take notice. Pay attention. What is your body communicating? Compression and contraction in your shoulders, stomach, and back can be a way of building resistance and feeling safe and secure. But fear and resistance—and the desire for safety and security—lead us to create a prison of our own making. Being with this recognition is much harder than knowing it intellectually.

In one of my workshops, a student I'll call Jeff spoke about an ache in his jaw and the white knuckles he frequently experienced. He was desperate to hold onto the money he had saved, fearful that it would somehow be taken away. He felt overwhelmed, spending his waking moments scheming for the future and trying to control his earnings, and sleepless nights riddled with anxiety. He began to feel sick, plagued by constant headaches, flu, and lower backache.

In our class, Jeff began to practice mindfulness, opening up to risk and sharing his fears with others. In return, he heard other students' stories of worry—financial worries, health worries, relationship worries—and he began to loosen. He saw how many of us suffer as we worry about the future. He decided to reach out to others and practice generosity, giving to a charity that spoke to his heart. Surprisingly, as he gave, he felt more abundant, generous, and connected to doing good in the world. As Jeff began to loosen his grip, to open his palms to give and receive, he began to feel into his rhythm of breathing, connecting him to the interconnected web of life. Rather than spending so much time in his head, scheming and planning, he began to relax into the notion that there is no controlling the future. Comfort and ease started to pulse through his body.

Transformation happens when we get out of the way and engage in the dance of life. Sometimes it's a limp, trudge, waltz, sometimes a rumba, and sometimes a slow and intimate sway. Once you accept that life is messy for everyone—that this is our shared humanity—it feels like awakening from a dream or a deep sleep. In the aliveness of authentic, human, vulnerable conversation, there is no going back to sleep. The cage that may have once felt safe and protective now feels claustrophobic and confining.

In that space, we each get to be in a real conversation together. There is no need to fix or try to solve a problem for another. Rather, listening and speaking in this reciprocal exchange is a blessing that is healing. The feeling of being heard and witnessed is a precious treasure. Being present with another is a gift, one that requires empty moments that are unplanned and able to be filled. When we are programmed from one goal to another, there is little time for the unknown to make itself known.

Open yourself to inclusivity, respect, and generosity. Self-compassion, kindness, wholeness, and doing good lead to feelings of belonging, love, and open-hearted generosity. Nurture your interconnected relationship with others and the world at large. Rather than having winners and losers, we can all feel valued and respected, finding our unique gifts and offering them through a generous heart. We are each part of the whole, creating a ripple effect of kindness and acceptance.

WEEK 8 INTENTIONS

During this week of the MBSE program, you will begin:

- To practice being kind to yourself. Self-compassion is not a selfish act: it has ripples that go far and wide into the world. You start with yourself.

- To embrace the fullness of your life, whatever the landscape. Notice the stress you feel when you hold onto expectations and judgments of how you want things to be. Exhale into things as they are and dance with what is. You may find that when you loosen your grip, surprising gifts can be found in disappointments and in letting go.

- To feel into our shared human experience of being alive. We all share the experiences of disappointment, difficulty, and loss as well as joy, gratitude, and well-being. We all are interconnected, a common thread joining our lives, breath by breath, moment by moment.

WEEK 8 DAILY PRACTICE

The list below details your practice for week 8. Read through it and, if you like, use it to prepare in advance for the week's practice. You can download a printable version of this list at https://www.newhar binger.com/44932 and post it in a place where you can see it easily. Visit the same URL to download the Art of Mindfulness Practice Guide, which contains directions for the body scan, sitting meditation, and gentle stretching yoga. Audio guides for these practices are available there, too.

1. Try one of the week 8 Mindful Art Encounters every day.

2. Each day, practice thirty minutes of sitting meditation, gentle stretching yoga, walking meditation, or body scan. You can also combine a few practices—for example, ten minutes of yoga followed by ten minutes of a sitting meditation. Or start with an awareness of breath breath meditation (part of the sitting meditation found in the online practice guide) for ten minutes and then follow it with a ten- to fifteen-minute body scan or a ten-minute loving-kindness meditation. Experiment. See what practices resonate, but be sure to plan and schedule the time so you continue with a regular daily practice. You are beginning to create a practice that works for you. If going without recordings feels too difficult, alternate days using recordings with days of going without.

3. When you are not doing the above formal practices, practice informal mindfulness by being as aware and awake as possible throughout the day.

4. Bring awareness to all of your interpersonal interactions and communications. Pause; then be present to the person in front of you and to yourself.

5. Begin to create a life you love. This is your life, being created moment to moment. The art of living is the most profound work of art that you can create. Start to mindfully create a life filled with intention, practice (both formal and informal), art encounters, and journaling. Practice intention with what you say yes and no to.

6. Every day this week (or as often as you can), go outside to connect to nature, breathing in the flora and fauna. Feel the support of the ground as you walk, connecting you to all living things. Sense into a feeling of belonging to this beautiful world. Bring awareness to feeling the breeze on your face, how it touches your skin and whether it's cool or warm. As you breathe, feel how air rhythmically flows into and then out of your body, touching and meeting the surrounding air. Feel and sense the air feeding and nourishing all the cells in your body and mind, how it circulates within your bloodstream and organs, and how it is essential to your well-being. Take in the energy of air on the inhalation and the release of air on the exhalation and feel the miracle of how this all automatically functions without you having to do anything, and how the same process is present in plants, animals, and birds. It is a dance of life magically moving and transforming, moment to moment.

7. Complete the Reflecting on the Week section at the end of this chapter.

Mindful Art Encounter #27: Being the Wind

Materials: Paper, art materials of your choice, pen or pencil, journal

Note: Before starting this exercise, review the guide for the sitting meditation in the online practice guide.

Begin by doing a five-minute sitting meditation. When you are finished, gather your art materials. Feeling into your body, begin to draw the sensation of wind, of the movement of air as it enters and leaves the body. How can you express the feeling of being filled with and then emptied of the air that we all share?

Begin making marks without too much thinking or planning. Just express movement, flow, and the sense of air. Are you feeling more familiar with this creative process now, at this point in your journey? Does it feel playful, exciting, and fresh?

When you have completed the drawing, place your crayon or pencil down. Close your eyes and feel what is to be felt. What do you feel in your body? Is there a new awareness?

Stand up and stretch your arms above your head. Reach as high has you can and then use movement to express the feeling of wind. Bend and stretch, step and lunge, allow your arms to move slowly and quickly as the wind. Become the wind, play as the wind. You are taking the experience of visual expression from two dimensions into time and space, moving in three dimensions.

After a few minutes, stop. Close your eyes and sense into the sensations in the body. Are you experiencing judgment, discomfort, pain, stiffness, anything that you may not have been aware of before?

Any time you do this exercise, journal about your experience.

Mindful Art Encounter #28: Being the Ocean

Materials: Paper, art materials of your choice, pen or pencil, journal

Note: Before starting this exercise, review the guide for the loving-kindness meditation found in the downloadable Art of Mindfulness Practice Guide found at http://www.newharbinger.com/44932.

Begin with a five-minute loving-kindness meditation. If you are inspired, place one hand on your heart and repeat the following words throughout your meditation:

May I be happy.

May I be peaceful.

May I be safe and protected.

May I live with ease.

When you are finished, take three deep breaths. How do you feel after saying these words?

Close your eyes and bring to mind the ocean. Feel into the waves large and small, tides, currents, surf, rhythm and stillness, light reflecting on the water, reflections dancing and moving in a glistening dance of light and shadow, movement and stillness.

Gather your paper and art materials. Choose colors that you are inspired by and make gestures of shapes, curves, waves, and stillness. Express the ocean though gestures, marks, and color that tell a story of the ocean in all of its stages of emerging and submerging.

Begin to notice the tension revealed in the embrace of dark and light. You can interpret this dark and light in color, gesture, shapes, marks, or any way you are inspired to. The most important thing is to play, to let go of judgments that try to creep in. Before they take hold, bring awareness to the judging voice. Acknowledge that it is there and then ask it to take a walk and disappear.

Draw your unique interpretation of the ocean and the ocean within. What parts resonate with you, and what parts scare you? How does the water move? What is the temperature? Is it deep and clear, filled with garbage, or full of fish and other life? How could you convey "ocean" to an alien from Mars who had no idea what an ocean was? How can you convey the feeling, sensation, and experience of the ocean?

What is the ocean of your life right now? Is it still and glistening or rough, treacherous, and scary? Do you trust the tide, going in and going out in a natural rhythm? Or are you exhausted from swimming against the tide, treading water, drowning?

When a large wave comes, do you dive into it or try to dodge it? Do you feel afraid and anxious, or do you trust the process of riding the wave and feel safe, even with its height and force? When the water is still and glistening in the sun, are you able to surrender and float, enjoying the feeling of immersion?

When you splash around, do you enjoy the splash or prefer not to be splashed? Are you afraid of sharks and other fish? How deep are you willing to go? When the water is clear and still, can you dive down to see life below the water? Can you see the magic of another world making itself known and welcoming you with one surprise after another?

Draw the feeling of the ocean deep inside your body. You may want to draw the waves, the currents, the splashes, the tides, the place where the ocean meets the horizon, the glistening in the sunlight, the darkness during a storm, the water at night, the stars and moon reflected on its surface, the rhythm of the waves as they break and recess, forward and back, small and large in their waviness.

There are no right ways or wrong ways to do this. Embrace your way. Listen deeply to your intuition and let it guide you—no apologies, no excuses, no playing it small. Try not to replicate something you have seen that has been the expression done by another person. Tap into your deepest feeling about the ocean and, from this place, create a visual. Your interpretation of the ocean is unique, so take risks as you dive into the wellspring of your innate expression. Remember to embrace not only the light and beauty of the ocean, but also the dark and ugly side, too.

If you make a mess, which is advisable because it invites freedom of expression, make a big mess. Make an ugly drawing. Be bold rather than tentative. You can always layer, erase, and change; the process of experimentation leads to a richness of surface that tells a history of your process, your struggle, your willingness to risk and experiment, to fall down six times and get up seven. Most of us do not want to feel worthless, inadequate, or any such negative connotations. Let these feelings be. Allow yourself to feel vulnerable and open. Within this place lies growth, transformation, and surprises along your creative way.

Make mistakes and then turn them into something else. Nothing is beyond transformation. Everything is workable. Transform what you feel is a mess into a meaningful lesson. Transform anything into something else. Cover, cut, erase, draw on top of, glue, collage, tear, destroy. Let go of any attachment to how you *want* it to be and open yourself to possibility. Play with the process. Be okay with feeling lost, with doubt and failure. Just keep creating.

Be in the field of "not knowing." This is a place for surprise and new inspirations to be born. Without space, nothing can enter. Things change constantly. Be open to see the surprises that appear without you having to do anything, with less effort and more flow, emergence, surprise. Each time you let go, you are adding another level of exploration, rich with investigation and curiosity.

After you've finished your artwork, if you have the opportunity to be by the ocean, take time to sit alone at the water's edge. Take in the smells, the light, the patterns, the movement, the rhythm, the effortless coming and going of the waves, the sand at the edge of the water, the colors and shapes being transformed moment by moment, the stillness and agitation, the ebb and flow, the flotsam and jetsam, the waves becoming the ocean and the ocean becoming the waves.

Think of five things that you would like to give up and throw into the ocean. Write the list on leaves or organic paper, tear each item out, and fold it into little pieces. Stand at the edge of the ocean and throw each piece in. Let it go and breathe into the release. This ritual is powerful. If you cannot be at the ocean, find a special place in nature that speaks to you. Visualize the ocean and then release the papers into the earth or whatever is available to you at that time.

Any time you do this exercise, journal about your experience.

Mindful Art Encounter #29: Being the River

Materials: Paper, art materials of your choice, pen or pencil, journal

Take three deep breaths and visualize a river. Recall the feelings and the sensations you have felt while at a river's edge or maybe seeing a river in a movie or a photograph. Feel into the sound of the river gushing by after a storm or when it is still and reflecting the trees and vegetation along its banks. Is it gurgling, perhaps, like a brook? Hear the detour as the water meets a rock and naturally flows around it.

Feel into the banks on either side of the river. Do they feel like a container or a holding place or confining and restrictive? The river flows in its "river-ness." It does not try to be an ocean. It does its natural thing as it flows and moves around. Sometimes it forms puddles; sometimes it is still and quiet; other times it's noisy. It has ripples, waves, maybe a waterfall as it drops to another level.

Use your art materials to express the feeling of a river flowing. How can you express the feelings of "water-ness," "river-ness," flowing, reflecting, being still, moving, gushing, pooling, and so on? Let one mark inform the next and the next, and keep going, with marks and shapes that remind you of water, emulate water, and express your interpretation of a river and how being a river feels.

When you have completed your drawing, take some time to observe and really *see* the visual expression of river. How did this exercise feel? What thoughts, emotions, and sensations did it bring up for you? Were you surprised at your drawing?

Any time you do this exercise, journal about your experience.

Mindful Art Encounter #30: Being the Sky

Materials: Paper, art materials of your choice, pen or pencil, journal

Begin with a formal practice of your choice for five minutes. When you are finished, open your eyes and feel into your sensations, emotions, thoughts, and feelings.

Allowing yourself to feel into the spaciousness of the big blue sky, ask yourself: Does spaciousness frighten you? Or do you like the openness in which possibility can be born? Feel into the blueness, the vastness, the clouds (if there are any), the light and dark, and the place where the sky seems to end. Is it an end or just a beginning? How do you feel as you feel into the "sky-ness" inside your being?

Begin drawing your expression of "sky-ness." Imagine that you are trying to communicate this feeling of sky to a being from underground. Express what "sky" feels like to you. Begin to make marks and shapes and forms, using lines, dots, and anything you are inspired to use. You can tear, rip, color, erase, overlap and glue together, pull apart, collage. Your sky can house clouds, a rainbow, stars, the moon, the sun, light and dark, blues that feel heavy and thick and sometimes mystical, thunder and lightning, rain, wind, birds, fog, shades of blue, pink, yellow, green, violet, orange, and purple.

After ten minutes, place your materials down and close your eyes. Feel into your body as you experience how you are feeling after this encounter.

As your days and nights unfold, take moments to observe the sky. See how it changes moment to moment. What do you observe that surprises you? Really look and take in the feeling of sky. See the edge and how it meets the horizon. Is the sky wide and vast, or are you only seeing a small portion?

Any time you do this exercise, journal about your experience.

Mindful Art Encounter #31: Being a Tree

Materials: Paper, art materials of your choice, pen or pencil, journal

Imagine a tree as a metaphor for yourself. What kind of tree are you? How wide is your trunk? How tall are your branches? Do you have leaves or no leaves? How far do the branches reach up and spread out? Or is the tree mostly upright?

Gather your art materials and draw your tree. Are there branches, leaves, flowers, blossoms, a tree house? Whatever else you feel in your "tree-ness," describe it visually. Each branch can carry a message, a reminder of gifts to include in your daily practice. As some of the leaves fall, what do they represent? How can you express this letting go? What is included in the new growth?

Any time you do this exercise, journal about your experience.

Mindful Art Encounter #32: Conversation Drawing with Community

Materials: Two large rolls of paper, selection of pencils (soft and hard), black markers (thin, medium, and broad), crayons, ink, paper towels or napkins, glue; pen or pencil; journal

In week 1, you did a conversation drawing with yourself, and in week 6, you added a partner. This time, invite a larger group into a collaborative conversation. Honoring the way your unique voice comes together with the voices of others is a way to stand in your own shoes while also standing with others, creating a community of kind acceptance, diversity, and inclusion.

Part 1

Roll out the first paper on the floor or a table and place the art materials within easy reach. Ask each person to take a position around the paper. It might be helpful to agree on a time limit or other stopping point in advance.

Ask everyone to close their eyes or lower their gaze and take three deep breaths. Feel the sensations of the inhalation and exhalation in your own particular rhythm. Feel into the experience of breathing the shared air together. Ask the group to set the intention to be present and listen deeply to the experience of community and equality, and to feel into body sensations in all colors and dimensions of tightness, expansion, and restriction. Note that this exercise is done in silence. It is about listening deeply to what is being said nonverbally in the moment by each participant and requires full attention so you can respond with presence and intuition.

Ask everyone to make a mark—any mark—anywhere on the large sheet of paper, then continue mark-making in a free and playful way. Use lines of any length and width, dots of any size and distance apart, shapes of any size and form, words, images, abstracts, symbols, forms, and textures. Position your marks anywhere on the paper, feel free to change marks and lines made by others, and change position around the paper when desired. You can use an eraser to smudge marks or even erase them completely. Introduce any other means and variation of marks that come out of spontaneity as you express your authentic mark. Try not to be precious about what you have drawn or your ideas of how it should unfold. Stay aware of the breath, playing with self-discovery as well as the discovery of working with others.

Mark by mark, a collaborative expression, or conversation, will emerge on the paper, bringing together each voice as an equal and important part of the whole. There is no plan, no goal, no hierarchy, and no preconceived idea. You are each simply communicating to yourself and others who you are in this moment as you follow the thread one mark at a time, staying open to risk and surprise and engaging playfully, imaginatively, and creatively. If fear does arise, befriend it, investigate it, and find your new relationship to fear.

This process requires presence in each moment, engaging a quality of aliveness and process. It is not tethered to comparing, remembering, or habits, instead calling you to see things as if for the very first time, fully engaged. This requires being brave and willing to make mistakes. It invites you to be like a child again. You will fall down a lot. You will learn to get up and start again. Through this process of risking, sometimes making mistakes but always feeling alive, you will feel a sense of vulnerability within and with your community. You are sharing and dancing together in this music that is being composed.

Each person will be drawn to different ways of experimenting and creating. As the process unfolds, become aware of judgments about what you or others are drawing: *That's ugly. I've messed up. They've messed up. This is out of control. I prefer to work on my own. I'm not creative. They are not creative. I do not like this collaborative drawing.* As human beings, we have preferences; we like and dislike. Bring awareness to constant judgments. Can you feel okay with "what is" even when you don't like it? Remember, there is no right way or wrong way to create the drawing. There is only your authentic engagement as you express and allow others to express your unique creative voices. Let go of needing things to be a certain way.

As you continue, what do you notice? Are you able to accept your and others' expressions even when you do not like them? Is the conversation inviting and spacious, or closed and filled with opinions and suggestions that are arising out of habits and familiar territory? Is your experience open or contracted? Are you exerting effort, pushing and striving, or are you allowing your marks to be freely drawn? Are you sensing a connection between your mark-making and the mark-making of others, and your inhalation and exhalation and theirs, feeling that you are all breathing and creating together, dissolving boundaries and coming together in inspiration and creativity?

When you reach the agreed-upon stopping point, place your media down. Ask everyone to close their eyes and take three deep breaths, feeling the breath in their body. Open your eyes and quietly observe the completed drawing, seeing how the different marks and media relate. Notice what the drawing is saying. Ask two people to hold up the drawing while the others gather in front and discuss the experience and what each person learned about him- or herself and the process of working with others.

Part 2

As a group, rip up the drawing. Tear it into as many pieces as you wish.

Feel into the sense of destruction, loss, and having to let go of something that you may have felt connected to. Is there resistance? Sadness? Anger? Or is there a sense of surprise, surrender, and an opening to new possibility? There may be a feeling of wild abandon and excitement, of letting go. How do you feel as you continue ripping and as the drawing becomes less and less recognizable?

When you've finished ripping, ask everyone to put the pieces down. Take three deep breaths. Close your eyes and feel what is to be felt in the body. Take a few more deep breaths. What thoughts, feelings, and sensations are you experiencing now? Notice judgment and allow the experience to be exactly as it is. There is no need to change anything.

Open your eyes. Do you see anything new?

Part 3

Roll out the second piece of paper and, once again working as a group, move the pieces around on the new paper, playing with their relationships to one another. Try placing them overlapping, close to each other, far apart, interwoven, joined, grouped, clustered, parallel, angled, diagonal, vertical, horizontal, tightly connected, with some folded to create three-dimensional forms, falling off the paper, hidden, revealed, simplified, divided, united, with space in between. Experiment. Begin to see how, moment to moment, the pieces form a new composition.

Explore relationships as you each begin gluing the pieces onto the new paper. Are there any surprises or fresh inspirations? Slowly let go of the old creation as it begins to fade into the past and a new composition emerges.

Ask two people to hold up the transformation with others gathered in front and share a discussion of the experience. This is a way to explore how we process loss in our community and how coming together and re-creating can be exhilarating and transformative as we witness a new creation being born.

After the group has left, ask yourself the following questions and write your answers below.

- How was it working with others? Do you prefer to work alone, or are you okay with risking and engaging in experimental play with others too?

- How did you feel about others changing your creative expression as it became part of the larger whole?

- What have you observed about the collaborative process? Did anything surprise you?

- What have you learned about yourself? Others? What do you share?

- How will this new perspective on community, diversity, and inclusivity inform your life going forward? What is it that you need to practice? What is it that you need to let go of?

_____

_____

_____

_____

_____

Any time you repeat this exercise, journal about your experience.

REFLECTING ON THE WEEK

When you finish the week's work, take some time to reflect before going on. Write in your journal or on the blank lines on whichever of the reflections or prompts below speak to you.

Reflections

- By accepting who you are, letting go of the need for external approval, and relaxing into life unfolding, you may experience your heart filling with compassion and kindness.

- Once you can freely tell your stories and give others the space to do the same, the walls that separate us begin to dissolve, and you may experience a sense of our shared humanity and our interconnected, living, breathing world.

- Meaningful, mindful connections expand the footprint of your life, deepening its richness and joy.

Journal Prompts

Write down your own reflections of this week. What discoveries did you make? Any ahas?

_____

_____

_____

_____

_____

_____

_____

_____

How can you be kinder to yourself?

_____

_____

_____

_____

What activities nourish you and inspire you to engage with life and feel alive?

_____

_____

_____

_____

What depletes you? How can you limit exposure to circumstances that drain and deplete you?

_____

_____

_____

_____

How can you begin to create clear boundaries as you take care of your well-being and sense of joy?

_____

_____

_____

_____

How can you commit to a daily routine of exercise and walking?

_____

_____

_____

_____

How can you practice self-compassion and loving-kindness as you walk through your life step by step? Remember, by working on yourself and becoming more mindful, you are in turn contributing to the well-being of others and our world. We are all interconnected.

_____

_____

_____

_____

As we approach the end of this program, I invite you to continue exploring your patterns, including those around endings. What is your relationship to endings? How do you feel when you hear the word "end"? Is sadness present? Do you feel excited for the ending to lead to a new beginning? How does this play out in your life?

_____

_____

_____

_____

_____

Who Am I Now?

For our life to be of value, I think we must develop basic human qualities—warmth, kindness, compassion. Then our life becomes meaningful and more peaceful—happier.

—14th Dalai Lama

Over the past eight weeks, you have been building a practice of meditation, both formal and informal, that you have integrated into your life. In this last week, you'll close the circle, coming back to the place where you began with new knowledge, new skills, new perceptions, and new ways to explore and investigate your life with a wider, kinder, and more open view. Who are you in this moment? What has changed with respect to how you relate to your life and others?

During your journey, you may have begun to let go of the closed perspective of "me," "mine," and "I" to see that we are all part of a much larger breathing, living whole. Ego causes a lot of suffering, and as you loosen the grip of everything revolving around *you* as the central point, you begin to feel a sense of freedom, connection, and kind consideration for the web of life. What we do to another, we do to ourselves, so the more generosity, love, and kindness we share, the happier we are. We begin to feel a sense of living in the flow.

You may also have learned that the greatest journey is back to your heart, deep inside where all the answers lie. When there is loving-kindness, self-compassion, and unconditional acceptance of yourself just as you are, without harsh judgments or wanting to be different, listening deeply to your intuition, instincts, and longings will guide you. The feeling of abundance allows you to be open and generous, rather than guarding and keeping what you have safe. There is enough—more than enough—of everything to go around. You may notice that the more open you are, the more you will receive.

This week, give thanks for the courage, strength, and willingness to look deeply at all aspects of yourself and come to a place of unconditional acceptance and love. You have been working toward this each week, and now you can begin to assimilate and digest the experience of self-acceptance, which is the inner strength that protects. This is not just the concept of self-acceptance, but the actual *feeling* that you

Creating Your Own Practice

Feel a sense of creativity and joyful play as you choreograph the exact practice that your body and intuition need right now. For example, you might create a practice that is like a relay race, with ten-minute segments that flow into each other, such as a ten-minute body scan, ten minutes of yoga, and then a ten-minute sitting practice with awareness of breath that then rolls right into your drawing encounters.

Are you in pain and discomfort or managing illness? If so, the body scan might be helpful with acceptance and compassion toward the body and ways of healing from within. Are you dealing with stressful relationships? A loving-kindness meditation could strengthen your sense of balance. Or how about a Mindful Art Encounter? If you'd like to release tension, try Freedom of Self-Expression (week 1). When things fall apart with illness or loss, Letting Go and Rebuilding, Part 1 may be helpful (week 2). Engage mindfully with your intuition as you call forth a practice that best serves the moment.

As a reminder, here are the formal practices you've learned, all of which have audio and print guides available at http://www.newharbinger.com/44932: body scan, gentle stretching yoga, sitting meditation (which includes choiceless awareness meditation), awareness of breath meditation, improvisational movement meditation, walking meditation, and loving-kindness meditation.

are okay: *I am okay. I am more than okay. I love all aspects of myself and know that I am valuable, creative, and willing to deepen my journey of life so I can feel more joy and use it to make a difference in the world.*

You have worked on facing your darkness and habits, on practicing seeing clearly, and your actions now come from this new view: *I am enjoying being less reactive and more engaged in present experience without expectation, judgments, or conditions.*

You are learning to engage with life from a point of intentionality, rather than guilt and wanting to please. You are learning to inhabit the place of "no" and to set boundaries to protect your well-being: *When I say yes or no, I mean it. I am empowered to take in only nourishing and loving content and act on things that are meaningful and important to me.*

You may begin to sense a feeling of balance, as well as an understanding of how to recognize when you are off-balance and what to do when this is felt: *I no longer feel like a victim and do not wish things to be different. I accept what is and simply redirect my focus and attention.*

Through the mindful art encounters, you are learning to be present in a creative way, letting the creative process (rather than a desire for a certain outcome) inform your words, actions, relationships, and work: *I am able to be present in a creative way. I listen deeply and respond to what is needed. Rather than advise or try to fix, I ask myself how I may serve the moment.*

Is this a doorway to a new way of being? Are you stepping though a doorway to your heart's longing, to what inspires you, to your feelings of connection, celebration, and gratitude for your life? When grounded in balance and acceptance, this can feel like coming home after a long journey of judging, contorting, and searching for answers outside. By choosing to be mindful, you are choosing to be radical in intention, vision, and action. Your practice will enhance your well-being, as well as that of your friends, family, and the world.

The journey is the destination. There are no goals to achieve. Sometimes, you might fall back into old ways and then beat yourself up for falling, so you essentially fall twice. Falling is part of the process. Bring kind awareness to those moments and then move on without digging deeper into negative reactivity. Yes, you will trip, and you will fall. The secret is to get up again and again, to begin again in each moment, doing your best, with the intention to be humble, vulnerable, and open. Continue on a path to mindfulness, creating your life as your greatest work of art. Everything is material for living life mindfully, compassionately, and kindly.

What brings you peace, and what pulls you away from it? Being able to discern this takes presence, practice, effort, and commitment. Anything worthwhile takes practice—and more practice. Make practice a part of your life. Everything is seamless: life, practice, intention, vision, joy, and well-being. Visualize your practice as planting and caring for seeds in the fertile, rich soil of your life. As you begin to water and nourish these new seeds, they will grow and blossom into a beautiful garden, enhancing and beautifying your world. I am planting seeds of kindness, creativity, trusting intuition, acceptance, gratitude, openness, surprise, breath, smiling, exercise, walking, and bathing. Which seeds will you plant?

WEEK 9 INTENTIONS

During this week of the MBSE program, you will begin:

- To become more comfortable with your own direction and personal practice, beginning to enjoy taking care of yourself and being responsible for your life: resilient, renewed, strong, self-aware, and free from outer harm.

- To play with the notions of pleasure, gratitude, and joy in being present. Feel the air on your skin, the miracle of your body sitting, sounds that surround you, and the light changing moment to moment.

- To befriend fear, take risks, and avoid going back to sleep, learning to enjoy the ride of ups and downs and going with the flow—the journey of your life.

- To be present as much of the time as possible. How often do you feel aligned with body, breath, and mind in the present moment? Throughout the day, ask yourself: Am I fully here now?

WEEK 9 DAILY PRACTICE

The list below details your practice for week 9. Read through it and, if you like, use it to prepare in advance for the week's practice. You can download a printable version of this list at http://www.newharbinger.com/44932 and post it in a place where you can see it easily.

1. Try one of the week 9 Mindful Art Encounters every day.

2. Using everything you have learned, create your own daily practice that you feel is best for you in this moment.

3. Practice mindful awareness of stress reactions and behaviors and notice how, with practice, you can respond to situations rather than react. Notice how you are tempering challenging situations and what skills you are calling upon in these moments.

4. Practice mindful awareness of feeling stuck, blocked, numb, or shut-off to the moment whenever it happens this week. Has this changed and become less stressful? Notice your relationship to circumstances, relationships, and communication with self and others. Has it changed? If so, how has it changed? What do you feel has been helpful?

5. Throughout the week, shake up your comfort zone and do things in new, even uncomfortable ways. If you take a particular route each day to work, take another route. Get lost and find your way back to familiar ground. If you hold your toothbrush in your right hand, change hands and see how it feels. Explore new materials, ways of being, and perspectives.

6. Throughout each day, do the three-breath practice (week 4) every hour. It is not easy to remember, but actually stop and take three breaths, being aware of your breathing.

7. Complete the Reflecting on the Week section at the end of this chapter.

Mindful Art Encounter #33: Mandala: The Heart of Being

Materials: Paper, a plate or other circular object just smaller than your paper to trace, art materials of your choice, pen or pencil, journal

In the Sanskrit language, "mandala" means a circle. A symbol of completion and wholeness, the mandala has been used as a source of reflection, healing, and vision for thousands of years by many cultures and religions, including by Buddhists, Navajo Native Americans, Romans, Greeks, Christians, Hindus, and Tibetans. Carl Jung, who used mandalas with patients, called them "a representation of the unconscious self."

Mandalas can be simple or complex. Often with a circle in the center, we see the same pattern in flowers blooming or in snowflakes.

Mandalas can be created like a meditation, and are traditionally used to reflect on harmony, wholeness, and life's journey. They remind us of the essence of our being and the wonder of life.

To begin this encounter, stand with your legs hip-width apart, arms at your sides, spine straight. Take three breaths and feel into the breath as it circles in and out of the body. Feel how the body receives this circle on the in-breath and returns it on the out-breath.

Slowly make five circles with your left arm, forward and back, keeping it straight and feeling into the shoulder. When you're finished, take a deep breath. Feel the sensations in the arm you just moved. Does it feel different from your right arm? Now make five circles with the right arm, forward and back. Is it easier on one side or the other?

Now gently make five little circles, or as many as feel right for you, with your head. Drop the head slightly forward, then move it to the right side, ear tilting toward your shoulder; then move your head slightly back to look up at the ceiling (but be careful not to bend the neck too far back), and to the left, with the left ear slightly moving toward the left shoulder. Next, reverse the movement to make five circles in the opposite direction. Pause and feel the sensations in your head, shoulders, neck, and anything else that you may be aware of.

Circle both shoulders: forward, then up toward the ears, then back, bringing the shoulder blades closer together, and then forward, up, and back. Repeat as many times as is right for you. Then reverse and move them in the opposite direction.

Circle the hips in whatever way feels comfortable. Bend your knees and keep them close together. This warms up the hip area.

Make circles with any part of the body that is calling for this movement. You are feeling into the form of a circle as you embody the movement. It is a smooth, flowing, and rhythmic movement that begins from your core. No matter what you are experiencing, this core is with you.

Next, gather your art materials to create a personal mandala. There is no right or wrong, good or bad outcome. It is an opportunity to reflect on your wholeness, inclusive of all of your parts. The mandala is meant to capture all of you.

Reflect on the various parts of your life: where you are right now and where you have been. Think about the big pictures of your life's journey. What are the key elements of "you"? We are each made up of attributes, qualities, aspirations, experiences, dreams, and memories.

To begin, use a plate or another circular object smaller than your paper to trace a large circle. This will be the outline of your mandala. Then draw a dot in the center of the circle.

Bring your attention to the dot. Feel into this tiny circle and bring the sensation of centering into your body. Feel the center or core of your body. The core is your strength, your place of balance and equilibrium. The center is the pelvis and the belly. All movement starts here.

Draw little circles around the dot, like the petals of a flower. Then, draw a circle around the outside of the petals as a border. I prefer to draw circles that are handmade and not exact, enjoying the playful way not-so-perfect circles add to the character of the mandala. Next, you might draw straight short lines around the circle, again adding dots and then encircling the pattern once again with a larger border circle.

Keep going, feeling into what you would like to do next. Explore the different patterns you can create with circles, large and small, and sizes in between. Draw them overlapping, joined, with spaces between, alternating small and large, and any other alternatives. Continue until you have reached the outer circle.

Now look at your mandala and see what you would like to add. Maybe color? Tone? Or perhaps you might fill in some of the shapes and leave others unfilled? This is a playful way of discovering patterns as you progress. You will be surprised and inspired as you go along.

When you're finished, answer the following questions on the lines below:

- As you created your mandala, was there a sense of acceptance, kindness, turning inward, and wholeness? Were you thinking much, or did you allow the mandala to emerge and be created as a meditation?

- What seems to be the message in the moment, communicated by the mandala?

- How are you feeling after the encounter? Were you surprised by your experience? What are you taking away from it?

- Some people feel a sense of wholeness and peace as they reflect on the image they created. Did you find this encounter relaxing?

_____

_____

_____

_____

_____

_____

_____

_____

_____

This activity can be woven into your regular meditation practice or simply returned to whenever you want to take time out and ground yourself in the moment.

Any time you repeat this exercise, journal about your experience.

Mindful Art Encounter #34: Planting Seeds, Growing Flowers

Materials: Paper, art materials of your choice, pen or pencil, journal

What flowers are seeding and blooming in the garden of your life? Are you tending your garden each and every day, watering the flowers with love, food, practice, and intention?

Tending the garden of your life with care and loving, kind attention may lead to understanding.

We have a choice as to what flowers we plant and water and how we choose to attend to them, knowing that as we feed them with loving-kindness, the results will be beautiful in some way.

Rather than feeling stuck in a garden that may have become overgrown with weeds, we can change the story and begin anew. Rather than thinking of them as "weeds," why not consider them as texture or wildflowers? They can still add to the overall beauty. My garden is wild and filled with flowers, bushes, trees, and weeds, and each adds its individual beauty to the natural flow of plants with different textures, different shades of green and other colors, and the way butterflies flit from one to another.

On a piece of paper, draw as many seeds as you would like to plant in the garden of your life. They can be different shapes and sizes and be at different levels below the ground.

Close your eyes and feel into the qualities and things that you would like to plant, tend to, water, and nourish. What would you like to see grow and flourish to enrich and enhance the garden of your life? For example, would you like to plant seeds of beauty, abundance, wisdom, practice, kindness, and joy? What seeds will grow your inner feelings of acceptance and "good enough"?

From the seeds, draw the stems and flowers that will grow. There are so many shapes to explore: flowers can be represented by circles, squares, triangles, or amorphous shapes. How does your garden grow? You can add a word or phrase in the center of a flower, on each petal, on the leaves, in the sky above, and maybe others in each seed. What will you nourish your garden with each day?

When you're finished, answer these questions on the lines provided.

What do you have to let go of to cultivate the environment for seeds of goodness to grow in your garden? What do you have to stay away from? For example: violent content in movies and television, unhealthy relationships, substances that numb, addiction to screens and phones, constant busyness, alcohol, shopping, unhealthy foods, not taking care of yourself, the need to be right, and so on.

_____

_____

_____

_____

_____

What do you need to invite more of to cultivate a nourishing environment for these seeds to grow?

_____

_____

_____

_____

Any time you do this exercise, journal about your experience.

Mindful Art Encounter #35: Who Am I Now?

Materials: Pencil or pen, journal

List twenty words answering the question: Who am I now? Try not to think too much. Avoid censoring or judging your words. Just list the qualities that come to you immediately, as if you were describing yourself to a stranger.

1. _____
2. _____
3. _____
4. _____
5. _____
6. _____
7. _____
8. _____
9. _____
10. _____

11. _____
12. _____
13. _____
14. _____
15. _____
16. _____
17. _____
18. _____
19. _____
20. _____

Now, look back at your answers to Mindful Art Encounter #1 (week 1). Has your knowing of who you are changed? If so, how? Have the practices changed you? How?

_____

_____

_____

_____

Any time you repeat this exercise, journal about your experience.

REFLECTING ON THE WEEK

When you finish the week's work, take some time to reflect before going on. Write in your journal or on the blank lines on whichever of the reflections or prompts below speak to you.

Reflections

- A mindful life of meaning, happiness, and resilience goes hand in hand with a formal practice that works with your life and the informal practice that *is* your life. They are not either-or or separate. They form one seamless practice that is ongoing, flowing from moment to moment.

- Mindful moments are all joined by presence, practice, and the power of discipline. Your practice isn't just another thing you have to do; rather, it is self-directed, inspired by taking care of yourself and knowing how it enhances your life. Befriend your practice as a lifelong commitment, nurturing the seeds of goodness in the garden of your life.

- To create your personal practice moving forward, engage mindfully with your life and call forth a practice that best serves your present moment.

Journal Prompts

Write down your own reflections of this week. Any ahas?

_____

_____

_____

_____

_____

_____

_____

_____

What is it that you need to invite into your daily practice? What would you like to let go of?

_____

_____

_____

_____

_____

What brought you to this workbook? What did you want to or hope would happen?

_____

_____

_____

_____

Why did you stay to the end of the course? What sacrifices did you make?

_____

_____

_____

What, if anything, did you receive? What did you learn about yourself?

_____

_____

_____

What obstacles did you encounter, and what did you learn about yourself in working through these obstacles?

_____

_____

_____

How do you feel about the program ending?

_____

_____

_____

What short-term goals do you have for including mindfulness and meditation in your daily life?

_____

_____

_____

What obstacles may stand in your way of reaching these goals? How will you keep the momentum of your practice going?

_____

_____

_____

_____

_____

Celebrating Each Moment:
Mindfulness for the Rest of Your Life

We are because I am. I am because we are.

—African proverb

Mindfulness is an experiential practice. It is not reading about and intellectualizing about being mindful. It is about rolling up your sleeves, getting dirty, and engaging in all experience—even that which is uncomfortable, difficult, and challenging. It is about being open to vulnerability and seeing all experience as part of the journey of life.

We practice mindfulness as the practice for life, and there are no shortcuts. Practice is cumulative. It is done every day. With practice, we might find that we become kinder and more patient. We look at things more openly. We are present. We are more resilient, better able to deal with stress, surprise, and loss, better prepared to adapt and go with the flow, less attached to outcomes. We can relax into life unfolding without expectations and judgments. We may notice that we are happier.

The work is to integrate what you have learned and stand firmly, grounded in that which you are. What are your values, intention, and vision for your life? What do you want to do with this one precious life—and how has your answer changed over the course of your journey? Do the inner work of creating, being, and expressing your authentic self beyond opinion, concept, and theory. Tell your story with the voice of honesty and trust your inner guidance. This can be powerful and freeing, and you begin to break the ties that bind.

As you come to the end of the book, how can your practice support you in your busy life? Are you an all-or-nothing person, or can you create a practice that will enhance your life rather than be another thing on your to-do list? Here are a few things to keep in mind as you move forward:

- Step out of "doing" mode and meet your practice from a different angle: one of stopping and taking care of yourself. Be with yourself in a kind and nurturing way, as you would do for a baby.

- Your breath is always there. It is your true friend.

- As you begin to see negativity and patterns that you may have previously been unaware of, practice with deep sincerity and the longing to learn and relate in new ways. The landscape is rich and full of gifts that mirror your inner dialogue. You are touching into your essence and making known what was hidden.

- There is no "good" practice or "bad" practice. There is only practice for practice's sake. To see clearly what is happening moment to moment and how you create your own suffering, to accept things as they are: that is practice.

- Every moment is a chance to begin again. Make a contract with yourself as you move into your new life: See the things that nurture you and fill you up and see the things that do not. Feel into the choices that are right for you experientially rather than intellectually.

- You are here now. This is the only moment you have, so allow thoughts, ideas, events, sensations, emotions, desires, and viewpoints to be.

- There is no fixed "self" and no "me, mine, or I." The image you have of yourself is an illusion, not to be believed. You are changing moment to moment, and you get to engage in each moment fully. This is the process of being alive and responding to life circumstances.

Life is a sacred journey. Understanding who you are from the core is a practice that prepares you for a meaningful, intentional, and magical journey over mountains and into valleys, lakes, oceans, clouds, and wide sky.

May your journey continue in beautiful and meaningful ways as your practice strengthens, and may you stay close to your intuition and what brings you back to your heart.

May you continue exploring, engaging curiosity, and embracing change with an open heart and mind, remaining open and vulnerable and inviting joy in the present moment. May you bring kind attention to each experience, even when you fall down and make mistakes.

May you continue creating and exploring marks of self-expression. May you stay close to a creative community or a group that shares the values of being creative and mindful, participate in retreats, and seek out inspiring mindfulness teachings in magazines, books, and elsewhere.

And may your practice be your trusted friend, with you through all your days for the rest of your life. May it color your life with the vibrancy of engaged presence in ordinary moments. May you befriend your breath, knowing that it is your anchor for life. May you attend to the breath with appreciation and kind attention. May you become intimate with your process of breathing as a beloved friend who is with you in every step.

> *Dear Ones,*
> *Be love,*
> *Be peace*
> *Be kind,*
> *Be true,*
> *Be now.*
> *With all my heart, thank you for your practice, beauty,*
> *courage, and creativity.*
>
> —Janet

Acknowledgments

To **Jon Kabat Zinn** for his teachings, inspired presence, and unconditional friendship.

To my **best friend, Silvia**: *An Artful Path to Mindfulness* was born from a broken heart—inspired by our friendship in Rivonia, South Africa, at the farm Shamballa.

To my beloved **parents**, Lily and Joe Slom, who gave me the gifts of life and unconditional love. Through their example I learned kindness—we are all ONE family on earth. Arthur Dunkelman, I am immensely grateful for your assistance and kind support. Sharing a practice and an adventure of art and mindfulness is a gift.

To my **beloved family**, Gina, Daniel, Lily, Zachary, and Dylan: you are my heart; love beyond time and space. Hours of fun drawing together have inspired this Artful Path. My brother Richard and his wife Priscilla, and nieces Mikayla, Myleigh, and Megan, for your loving support. Ashley S. for bringing our family to America, for all the precious moments, and for all the creative projects over the years.

My **beloved teachers**: Joe Slom, H. H. Dalai Lama, Jon Kabat-Zinn, Saki Santorelli, Sharon Salzberg, Pema Chödrön, Thich Nhat Hanh, Ekhart Tolle, Nelson Mandela, Chögyam Trungpa Rinpoche, Tara Brach, Jack Kornfield, Krishna Murti, Lynn Koerbel, Florence Meleo Meyer, Melissa Blacker, Joseph Goldstein, David White, Mary Oliver, and Rumi.

To each of my students throughout the years, love and deep appreciation for all that we shared and learned together. You have inspired this Artful Path to Mindfulness.

To Julie Mazur Tribe, your kindness and skilled editing have been a gift beyond words. My New Harbinger family: Elizabeth Hollis Hansen, for believing in my work and opening the door to New Harbinger; Gretel Hakanson, Jennifer Holder, Clancy Drake, Jesse Burson, Analis Souza, Amy Shoup, and Michele Waters. What a team! This has been a journey that I will hold in my heart forever. Your vision, editorial skills, marketing and creative expertise, and kind support have allowed this work to be born on the page so that it can be widely shared. Debra Annane, your presence, wisdom, and mindful guidance are within these pages. Immense gratitude.

Special thanks: Dr. Dale Atkins for your loving friendship and your most generous support of MBSE and *An Artful Path to Mindfulness*. Dale and Rob Rosen, deep gratitude for opening your hearts and home with a magical cottage where I could quietly write. Heather and Shephard Schwartz, for your love, generosity, support, and a lifetime of sharing. Orna and Geff Stern, for your love, generosity, and kindness. Your friendship is a blessing. An Artful Path began on Apache with Abigail and Cassie—playdates in the studio. Gabriella and Tucker Mays, for your warm welcome and support of my work, our inspired conversations, and precious times together. Jeff Elster, for your wisdom and kindness. Donatella Linari and Lenny Schwartz, for your kindness and shared adventures. Sylvia Atkins, for your generous and kind spirit, always creating connections. Steve and Wendy Siegel, for blessing my life and believing in my work and sharing your home and the magical cottage on the river where this Artful Path began. Lauren and Lakkie Kaplan, for a friendship that began in South Africa as children and continues to blossom in beautiful ways, and for your support of my work.

To **my beloved friends, colleagues, and family**. *An Artful Path to Mindfulness* is a record of precious shared moments that have inspired our hearts' journey through creative and mindful ways: Brenda G., Carol T., Mary Beth S., Debra A., Erika S., Alberto C., Rosemary W., Amy G., Amy S, .Kathy L., Dick B., Sandra B., Kiera M., Helen Z., Mrs. Penny, Bill A., Nina C. Q., Ann Marie N., Mary F., Sue S., Steve S., Wendy S., Mary H., Dan H., Nancy G., Jackie N., Raphael N., Carol P., Ruth S., Marvin S., Josephine J., Silvia R., Dorothy S., Suzanne A., Karl N., Elizabeth N., Virginia B., Chana G., Rabbi G., Dina K., Rabbi K., Rabbi W., Jill K., Philip E., Fanji M., Gene K., Gerard O.B., Frank P., Mandana P., Bobbie R., Lynn T., Julianna J., Sheldon H., Peppino S., Hymie L., Daniel M., Charles G., Rabbi R., Rev. S., Derek R., Laraine R., Doug M., Zayda V., Bob L., Bill H., Robin P., Melanie M., William S., Lisa I., David I., Jamie C., Glen C., Bonnie H., Dale H., Paul A., Myara B., Julie M., Charl M., Leslie C., Elizabeth O., Power B., Dr. Karen K., Don S., Paul S., Susanna C., Joe N., Harry C., Cindy R., Carol C., Gary C., Faith M., Bob M., Sandra L., Abigail S, Cassandra S., Stacy S., Liza, Simon, Lucie, Andries, Albanon, Jill D., Chuck E., Kelly M., Michael C., Devyani S., Raj G., Jack S., Tamsen G., Paul L., Pearl L., Stephanie B., Kay C., J. T., Amanda D., Frank D., Meryl M., Nanette G., Linda K., Jill D., D. J. C., Peter V. H., Carol D., Doug M. G., Pearl L., Celeste P., Jonathan M., and others. You know who you are. I am immensely grateful.

Throughout the years, my life has been blessed to have journeyed with each of you. Our connection is deep and my gratitude everlasting. Together we have shared a most precious journey

Thank you to my colleagues listed in this book's first few pages who have endorsed the book.

To the **artists past and present** who are living An Artful Path to Mindfulness—marking, creating their personal languages, genuine expressions, and embodiments of their vision—and whose intentions speak clearly through their self-expression: Brenda Goodman, Marina Abramovic, Louise Bourgeois, Marlene Dumas, Power Boothe, Susanna Coffey, Lynette Yiadome Boakye, Julie Mehretu, Helen Frankenthaler, Joan Mitchell, Cecily Brown, Charlene von Heyl, Yayoi Kusama, Hilma af Klint, Louise Bourgeois, Julie Mehretu, Agnes Martin, Wangechi Mutu, Dana Schutz, Barbara Kruger, Brice Marden, William Kentridge, Cy Twombly, Jackson Pollock, and Christopher Wool, to name just a few.

Practice Logs

Record of Mindful Moments

At least a few times this week, bring mindful awareness to an otherwise routine activity, such as washing the dishes, waiting in line, eating lunch, or walking from the car to your office. At the end of each day, see if you can recall at least one example of simple awareness. The first one has been done as an example. Download a blank PDF of this record at http://www.newharbinger.com/44932.

What was the situation? Where were you, who were you with, and what were you doing?	What feelings, thoughts, and sensations did you notice before you decided to experience this mindfully?	What feelings, thoughts, and sensations did you notice while doing this mindfully?	What did you learn from doing this?	What feelings, thoughts, and sensations are you noticing now as you write this?
Washing dishes after dinner	I was feeling hurried, shoulders and stomach tense, thinking, I wish Chris hadn't used so many dishes!	I felt the warm water on my hands and enjoyed seeing the dishes sparkle. Time seemed to stop for a moment.	Paying attention to physical sensations brings me into the here and now, and a loving task becomes more interesting.	Feeling the support of the chair I'm sitting on, the feel of the pen, and feeling thankful that a long day is over.

Pleasant Events Calendar

Use the following questions to focus your awareness on pleasant experiences as they are happening. Write down your observations later. The first column has been done as an example. Download a blank PDF of this form at http://www.newharbinger.com/44932.

Day of the week:	What was the experience?	Were you aware of the pleasant feelings while the event was happening?	How did your body feel, in detail, during this experience?	What moods, feelings, and thoughts accompanied this event?	What thoughts are in your mind now, as you write this down?
Sunday	Walk with dog	Yes	Energetic; comfortable in my skin	Feeling calm and peaceful	Fresh air always helps!

Adapted from *Full Catastrophe Living* by Jon Kabat-Zinn, PhD.

Unpleasant Events Calendar

Use the following questions to focus your awareness on unpleasant experiences as they are happening. Write down your observations later. The first column has been done as an example. Download a blank PDF of this form at http://www.newharbinger.com/44932.

Day of the week:	What was the experience?	Were you aware of the unpleasant feelings while the event was happening?	How did your body feel, in detail, during this experience?	What moods, feelings, and thoughts accompanied this event?	What thoughts are in your mind now, as you write this down?
Sunday	Getting stuck in traffic	Yes	Jaw tightening, breathing fast, hands clenched to steering wheel	Feeling angry at myself for not getting up in time, helpless	I'm going to remember to set my alarm.

Adapted from *Full Catastrophe Living* by Jon Kabat-Zinn, PhD.

Difficult Communications Calendar

This week, be aware of difficult or stressful communication *while it is happening.* At a later time, write about your experience in the chart below. Download a blank PDF of this form at http://www.newharbinger.com/44932.

Day of the week:	Describe the communication. With whom? What was the subject?	How did the difficulty come about?	What did you really want from the person or situation? What did you actually get?	What did the other person want? What did they actually get?	How did you feel during and after this time?	Has this issue been resolved? How might it be?

Adapted from *Full Catastrophe Living* by Jon Kabat-Zinn, PhD.

More Mindfulness Resources

MINDFULNESS PROGRAMS, ORGANIZATIONS, AND TEACHERS

University of Miami Mindfulness Research and Practice Initiative
www.umindfulness.as.miami.edu

Mindful Kids Miami
www.mindfulkidsmiami.org

Mindful Life Project
www.mindfullifeproject.org

Mindfulness Meditation Centers
https://mindfulnessmeditationcenters.com

Institute for Mindfulness South Africa
https://mindfulness.org.za/

Brown University School of Public Health Mindfulness Center
www.brown.edu/public-health/mindfulness/

UMass Medical School Center for Mindfulness
www.umassmed.edu/cfm/

Mind and Life Institute
www.mindandlife.org/

Omega Institute
www.eomega.org/

Kripalu
https://kripalu.org/

Insight Meditation Society
www.dharma.org/

Mindfulness-Based Cognitive Therapy
http://mbct.com/

Greater Good Science Center
https://greatergood.berkeley.edu/

Greater Good Magazine
https://ggsc.berkeley.edu/what_we_do/greater_good_magazine

Sharon Salzberg
www.sharonsalzberg.com

Bob Stahl
www.mindfulnessresources.com

Dr. Rick Hansen
www.rickhanson.net/

Shambhala
www.shambhala.com/

Dr. Kristin Neff
https://self-compassion.org/

Tara Brach
www.tarabrach.com/

Joseph Goldstein
www.1440.org/about

Dr. Sharon Theroux
www.mindfulsouthflorida.com

Dr. Valerie York Zimmerman
www.miamimindfulness.com

Saki Santorelli, Guest-House Educational Services

Open Center
www.opencenter.com

Janet Slom online:
www.MBSE.info
www.janetslom.com
Twitter: @janetslom
Facebook: Janet Slom

BOOKS

Aimone, Steven. 2009. *Expressive Drawing: A Practical Guide to Freeing the Artist Within* (Live and Learn Series AARP). New York: Lark Books.

Analayo. 2018. *Satipatthana Meditation: A Practice Guide*. Cambridge, UK: Windhorse Publications.

Ando, Erica. "William Kentridge: Five Themes." Utopian Studies 21, no. 2, 2010.

Andre, Christophe. 2016. *Looking at Mindfulness: Twenty-Five Paintings to Change the Way You Live*. New York: Blue Rider Press.

Augsburger, Esther K. 1978. "Paul Klee and Time." Southeastern College Art Conference Review 9, no. 3.

Austin, James H. 1998. *Zen and the Brain: Toward an Understanding of Meditation and Consciousness*. Cambridge, MA: MIT Press.

Bardache, Nancy. 2012. *Mindful Birthing*. New York: HarperCollins Publishers.

Bodi, Bhikku. 2000. *The Noble Eightfold Path*. Onalaska WA: Pariyatti Publishing.

Bolen, Jean Shinoda. 1999. *The Millionth Circle: How to Change Ourselves and the World—The Essential Guide to Women's Circles*. Berkeley, CA: Conari Press.

Brach, Tara. 2005. *Radical Self-Acceptance: A Buddhist Guide to Freeing Yourself from Shame*, audiobook. Boulder, CO: Sounds True.

Brach, Tara. 2013. *True Refuge: Finding Peace and Freedom in Your Own Awakened Heart*. New York: Bantam.

Brown, Brené. 2004. *Daring Greatly: How the Courage to Be Vulnerable Transforms the Way We Live, Love, Parent, and Lead*. New York: Gotham.

Brown, Brené. 2010. *The Gifts of Imperfection: Let Go of Who You Think You're Supposed to Be and Embrace Who You Are*. Center City, MN: Hazelden Publishing.

Buber, Martin. 1962. *I and Thou*, 2nd ed, trans. by Ronald Gregor Smith. New York: Charles Scribner's Sons.

Cameron, Julia. 1996. *Vein of Gold: A Journey to Your Creative Heart.* New York: Tarcher/Putnam.

Cameron, Julia. 1997. *The Artist's Way: A Course in Discovering and Recovering Your Creative Self.* New York: MacMillan.

Chase, Michael. 2017. *Mask: Making, Using, and Performing.* Stroud, Gloucestershire, UK: Hawthorn Press, Ltd.

Chidvilasananda, Swami. 1996. *The Yoga of Discipline.* New York: Soma Books, Ltd.

Chödrön, Pema. 1991. *Wisdom of No Escape.* Boston: Shambhala Publications, Inc.

Chödrön, Pema. 1994. *Start Where You Are: A Guide to Compassionate Living.* Boston: Shambhala Publications, Inc.

Chödrön, Pema. 1997. *When Things Fall Apart: Heart Advice for Difficult Times.* Boulder, CO: Shambhala Publications, Inc.

Chödrön, Pema. 2001. *The Places That Scare You: A Guide to Fearlessness in Difficult Times.* Boulder, CO: Shambhala Publications, Inc.

Dalai Lama. 1996. *Tibetan Portrait: The Power of Compassion.* New York: Rizzoli.

Dalai Lama. 2006. *How to See Yourself for Who You Really Are.* New York: Atria Books.

Davidson, Richard, and Anne Harrington. 2002. *Visions of Compassion.* New York: Oxford University Press.

Davidson, Richard J., and Sharon Begley. 2012. *The Emotional Life of Your Brain: How Its Unique Patterns Affect the Way You Think, Feel, and Live—and How You Can Change Them.* New York: Hudson Street Press.

Emerling, Jae. 2010. "Marina Abramovic: The Artist Is Present: Museum of Modem Art, New York: X-Ira." *Contemporary Art Quarterly* 13, no. 1.

Feldman, Christina. 2003. *Silence: How to Find Inner Peace in a Busy World.* Berkeley, CA: Rodmell Press.

Genii, Robert. "The Painter's Keys." *Paul Klee Art Quotes.* http://guote.robertgenn.com/auth search.php?.

Germer, Christopher. 2009. *The Mindful Path to Self-Compassion: Freeing Yourself from Destructive Thoughts and Emotions.* New York: The Guilford Press.

Germer, Christopher, and Kristin Neff. 2019. *Teaching the Mindful Self-Compassion Program: A Guide for Professionals.* New York: The Guilford Press.

Goldstein, Joseph. 2012. *Abiding in Mindfulness, Volume 2: On Feeling, the Mind, and Dhamma* (audiobook). Boulder, CO: Sounds True.

Habson, Richard, and Richard Mendius. 2009. *Buddha's Brain.* Oakland, CA: New Harbinger Publications.

Hayes, S. C. 2005. *Get Out of Your Mind and into Your Life: The New Acceptance and Commitment Therapy.* Oakland, CA: New Harbinger Publications.

Hayes, Steven C., Victoria M. Follette, and Marsha M. Linehan. 2011. *Mindfulness and Acceptance: Expanding the Cognitive-Behavioral Tradition*. New York: The Guilford Press.

Herbert, Martin. 2007. "Tina Bausch." *Modern Painters*, December 2006/January 2007.

Kabat-Zinn, Jon. 1990. *Full Catastrophe Living, Using the Wisdom of the Body and Mind to Face Stress, Pain, and Illness*. New York: Delacorte.

Kabat-Zinn, Jon. 1990. *Letting Everything Become Your Teacher: 100 Lessons in Mindfulness*. New York: Delta.

Kabat-Zinn, Jon. 1993. "Meditation." In *Healing and the Mind* by Bill Moyers. New York: Doubleday, 115–143.

Kabat-Zinn, Jon. 1994. *Wherever You Go, There You Are: Mindfulness Meditation in Everyday Life*. New York: Hyperion.

Kabat-Zinn, Jon. 2005. *Coming to Our Senses: Healing Ourselves and the World Through Mindfulness*. New York: Hyperion.

Kabat-Zinn, Jon. 2010. *Mindfulness for Beginners: Reclaiming the Present Moment—and Your Life*. Boulder, CO: Sounds True.

Kabat-Zinn, Myla, and Jon Kabat-Zinn. 2014. *Everyday Blessings: The Inner Work of Mindful Parenting*. New York: Machete Books.

Kant, Michelle Marder. 2006. "Modernism, Postmodernism, or Neither? A Fresh Look at 'Fine Art.'" *Arts Education Policy Review* 107, no. 5.

Klee, Paul. 1968. *The Diaries of Paul Klee, 1898–1918*. Berkeley, CA: University of California Press.

Knott, Robert. 1979. "Paul Klee and the Mystic Center." *Art Journal* 38, no. 2, 1978–1979.

Kornfield, Jack. 1995. *A Path with Heart: A Guide Through the Perils and Promises of Spiritual Life*. New York: Bantam.

London, Peter. 1989. *No More Secondhand Art: Awakening the Artist Within*. Boston: Shambhala Publications, Inc.

May, Rollo. 1982. *Courage to Create*. New York: Bantam Books.

McCown, Donald, et al. 2011. *Teaching Mindfulness: A Practical Guide for Clinicians and Educators*. New York: Springer.

Murti, Krishna, and D. Rajagopal. 1993. *Think On These Things*. New York: Harper & Row.

Nachmanovitch, Stephen. 1990. *Free Play: The Power of Improvisation in Life and the Arts*. New York: Penguin.

Nachmanovitch, Stephen. 2019. *The Art of Is: Improvising as a Way of Life*. Novato, CA: New World Library.

Naves, Mario. 2009. "Exhibition Notice: Marlene Dumas: Measuring Your Own Grave." *New Criterion* 27, no. 6.

Neff, Kristin. 2015. *Self-Compassion: The Proven Power of Being Kind to Yourself*. New York: William Morrow.

Neff, Kristin. 2018. *The Mindful Self-Compassion Workbook: A Proven Way to Accept Yourself, Build Inner Strength, and Thrive*. New York: The Guilford Press.

Nhat Hanh, Thich. 1976. *The Miracle of Mindfulness*. Boston: Beacon Press.

Nhat Hanh, Thich. 1998. *The Heart of the Buddha's Teaching: Transforming Suffering into Peace, Joy & Liberation: The Four Noble Truths, the Noble Eightfold Path & Other Basic Buddhist Teachings*. Berkeley, CA: Parallax Press.

Nhat Hanh, Thich. 2014. *How to Sit, Mindfulness Essentials*. Berkeley, CA: Parallax Press.

Nhat Hanh, Thich. 2015. *How to Love, Mindfulness Essentials*. Berkeley, CA: Parallax Press.

Nhat Hanh, Thich. 2015. *No Mud No Lotus: The Art of Transforming Suffering*. Berkeley, CA: Parallax Press

Oliver, Mary. 1986. *Dream Work*. New York: Atlantic Monthly Press.

Oliver, Mary. 2005. *Why I Wake Early: New Poems*. Boston: Beacon Press.

Oliver, Mary. 2016. *Blue Horses: Poems*. New York: Penguin Books.

O'Reilly, Sally. 2008. "William Kentridge: Ways of Seeing." *Art Review* 21.

Palmer, Parker J. 2005. *The Politics of the Brokenheart*. Kalamazoo, MI: Fetzer Institute.

Rogers, Holly, and Margaret Maytan. 2012. *Mindfulness for the Next Generation: Helping Emerging Adults Manage Stress and Lead Healthier Lives*. Oxford, UK: Oxford University Press.

Saitzyk, Steven L. 2013. *Place Your Thoughts Here: Meditation for the Creative Mind*. Minneapolis: First Thought Press.

Salesman, Amy. 2014. *A Still Quiet Place: A Mindfulness Program for Teaching Children and Adolescents to Ease Stress and Difficult Emotions*. Oakland, CA: New Harbinger Publications.

Saltz, Jerry. 2018. "How to Be an Artist: 33 Rules to Take You from Clueless Amateur to Generational Talent (or at Least Help You Live Life a Little More Creatively)." *Vulture Magazine* 27, November.

Salzberg, Sharon. 1995. *Loving-Kindness: The Revolutionary Art of Happiness*. Boston: Shambhala Publications, Inc.

Salzberg, Sharon. 1997. *A Heart as Wide as the World*. Boulder, CO: Shambhala Publications, Inc.

Salzberg, Sharon. 2002. *Faith: Trusting Your Own Deepest Experience*. New York: Riverhead Books.

Salzberg, Sharon. 2013. *Real Happiness at Work: Meditations for Accomplishment, Achievement, and Peace*. New York: Workman Publishing Company.

Santorelli, Saki. 1999. *Heal Thy Self: Lessons on Mindfulness in Medicine*. New York: Three Rivers Press.

Schumacher, Rainald. 2009. "Marlene Dumas." *Flash Art, International Edition* 42.

Shapiro, Shauna L., and Linda E. Carson. 2009. *The Art and Science of Mindfulness: Integrating Mindfulness into Psychology and the Helping Professions*. Washington, DC: American Psychological Association.

Suzuki, Shunru. 1970. *Zen Mind, Beginner's Mind*. New York: Weatherhill.

Spector, Jack. 1998. "The State of Psychoanalytic Research in Art History." *The Art Bulletin* 70, no. 1.

Stahl, Bob. 2014. *Mindfulness-Based Stress Reduction Workbook for Anxiety*. Oakland CA: New Harbinger Publications.

Stahl, Bob, and Elisha Goldstein. 2010. *A Mindfulness-Based Stress Reduction Education Workbook*. Oakland, CA: New Harbinger Publications.

Stahl, Bob, and Goldstein, Elisha. 2015. *MBSR Every Day: Daily Practices from the Heart of Mindfulness-Based Stress Reduction*. Oakland, CA: New Harbinger Publications.

Sterckx, Pierre. 2000. "Bringing Out the Primitive." *Art Press* 257, May.

Storr, Robert. 1986. *Philip Guston, Modern Masters Series*, vol. 11. New York, Abbeville Press.

Trungpa, Chögyam. 1984. *Shambhala: Sacred Path of the Warrior*. Boulder, CO: Shambhala Publications, Inc.

Trungpa, Chögyam. 2008. *True Perception: The Path of Dharma Art*. Boulder, CO: Shambhala Publications, Inc.

Turner, Christopher. 2010. "Through the Eyes of a Child." *Tate Etc* 19.

Vesely, Dalibor. 2011. "Surrealism and the Latent World of Creativity." *Art* 59, no. 3.

Weschler, Lawrence, and Robert Irwin. 2009. *Seeing Is Forgetting the Name of the Thing One Sees: Over Thirty Years of Conversations*. Berkeley, CA: University of California Press.

Willard, Christopher, and Amy Saltzman. 2017. *Teaching Mindfulness Skills to Kids and Teens*. New York: The Guilford Press.

Williams, Mark, et al. 2007. *The Mindfulness Way Through Depression: Freeing Yourself from Chronic Unhappiness*. New York: The Guilford Press.

References

Anderson, B. 2018. *Real Life Mindfulness: Meditations for a Calm and Quiet Mind.* Miami, FL: Mango Publishing.

Arrien, A. 1992. *The Four-Fold Way: Walking the Paths of the Warrior, Teacher, Healer, and Visionary.* New York: HarperCollins Publishers.

Chödrön, P. 2016. *When Things Fall Apart: Heart Advice for Difficult Times.* Boulder, CO: Shambhala Publications, Inc.

Donne, J. 1987. *Devotions Upon Emergent Occasions.* New York: Oxford University Press.

Eliot, T. S. 1963. *Collected Poems, 1909–1962.* New York: Harcourt Brace & Company.

Epictetus. 1994. *The Art of Living: The Classical Manual on Virtue, Happiness, and Effectiveness,* trans. Sharon Lebell. New York: HarperCollins Publishers.

Kabat-Zinn, J. 1994. *Wherever You Go There, You Are: Mindfulness Meditation in Everyday Life.* New York: Hyperion.

Kabat-Zinn, J. 2013. *Full Catastrophe Living, Revised Edition: How to Cope with Stress, Pain, and Illness Using Mindfulness Meditation.* New York: Piatkus Books.

Kabat-Zinn, J. 2013. *Mindfulness for Beginners: Reclaiming the Present Moment—and Your Life.* New York: Hachette Books.

Kabat-Zinn, J. 2018. *Falling Awake: How to Practice Mindfulness in Everyday Life,* New York: Hachette Books.

Kabat-Zinn, J. 2018. *The Healing Power of Mindfulness: A New Way of Being.* New York: Hachette Books.

Kabat-Zinn, J. 2018. *Meditation Is Not What You Think: Mindfulness and Why It Is So Important.* New York: Piatkus Books.

Mitschering, J., and Fairfield, P. 2019. *Artistic Creation: A Phenomenological Account.* Lanham, MD: Lexington Books.

Nachmanovitch, S. 1990. *Free Play: Improvisation in Life and Art.* New York: Penguin Putnam, Inc.

Nachmanovitch, S. 2019. *The Art of Is: Improvising as a Way of Life.* Novato, CA: New World Library.

Rilke, R. Maria. 1984. *Letters to a Young Poet,* trans. Stephen Mitchell. New York: Random House.

Rilke, R. Maria. 1994. *Rilke on Love and Other Difficulties: Translations and Considerations by John L. Mood,* trans. John L. Mood. New York: W. W. Norton & Co.

Rosenberg, M. 2015. *Nonviolent Communication: A Language of Life,* 3rd ed. Encinitas, CA: PuddleDancer Press.

Rumi, J. 1995. *The Essential Rumi,* trans. by Coleman Barks and John Moyne. New York: HarperCollins Publishers.

Rumi, J. 2017. *Love: The Joy that Wounds: The Love Poems of Rumi,* London: Souvenir Press.

Seka, M. I. 2014. *Life Lessons of Wisdom & Motivation: Volume I.* Scotts Valley, CA: CreateSpace Independent Publishing Platform.

Snel, E. 2013. *Sitting Still Like a Frog: Mindfulness Exercises for Kids (and Their Parents).* Boulder, CO: Shambhala Publications, Inc.

Stahl, B., and Goldstein, E. 2010. *A Mindfulness-Based Stress Reduction Workbook.* Oakland, CA: New Harbinger Publications.

Tolle, E. 2005. *A New Earth: Awakening to Your Life's Purpose.* New York: Dutton.

Winnicott, D. 1991. *Playing and Reality.* London: Psychology Press.

Janet Slom, MFA, is an artist, author, educator, and social entrepreneur who serves on the faculty at Lehigh University's Global Village, and as adjunct faculty for fourteen years at the Center for Mindfulness at the University of Massachusetts Medical School. She is founder of mindfulness-based self-expression (MBSE)—evolved from Jon Kabat-Zinn's mindfulness-based stress reduction (MBSR) program—which instructs students through an experiential curriculum to integrate mindfulness meditation, creativity through art, and mind-body practices into personal growth, mastery of one's professional field, and improvement of overall wellness. Originally from South Africa, her art installations have been exhibited throughout the globe.

Foreword writer **Jon Kabat-Zinn, PhD,** is internationally known for his work as a scientist, writer, and meditation teacher engaged in bringing mindfulness into the mainstream of medicine and society. He is professor of medicine emeritus at the University of Massachusetts Medical School; and author of numerous books, including *Full Catastrophe Living, Arriving at Your Own Door,* and *Coming to Our Senses.*

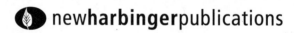

MORE BOOKS *from*
NEW HARBINGER PUBLICATIONS

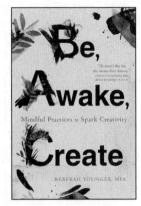

BE. AWAKE. CREATE
Mindful Practices to Spark Creativity
978-1684032389 / US $19.95

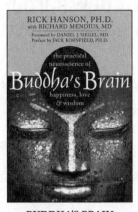

BUDDHA'S BRAIN
The Practical Neuroscience of
Happiness, Love & Wisdom
978-1572246959 / US $18.95

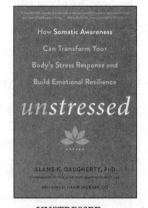

UNSTRESSED
How Somatic Awareness Can
Transform Your Body's Stress Response
& Build Emotional Resilience
978-1684032839 / US $16.95

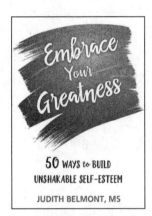

EMBRACE YOUR GREATNESS
Fifty Ways to Build
Unshakable Self-Esteem
978-1684032204 / US $16.95

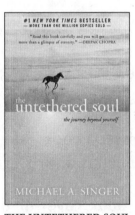

THE UNTETHERED SOUL
The Journey Beyond Yourself
978-1572245372 / US $17.95

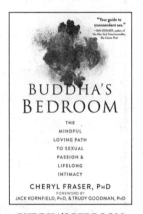

BUDDHA'S BEDROOM
The Mindful Loving Path to Sexual
Passion & Lifelong Intimacy
978-1684031184 / US $16.95

newharbingerpublications
1-800-748-6273 / newharbinger.com

(VISA, MC, AMEX / prices subject to change without notice)

Follow Us

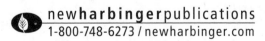

Register your **new harbinger** titles for additional benefits!

When you register your **new harbinger** title—purchased in any format, from any source—you get access to benefits like the following:

- Downloadable accessories like printable worksheets and extra content
- Instructional videos and audio files
- Information about updates, corrections, and new editions

Not every title has accessories, but we're adding new material all the time.

Access free accessories in 3 easy steps:

1. Sign in at NewHarbinger.com (or **register** to create an account).

2. Click on **register a book**. Search for your title and click the **register** button when it appears.

3. Click on the **book cover or title** to go to its details page. Click on **accessories** to view and access files.

That's all there is to it!

If you need help, visit:

NewHarbinger.com/accessories

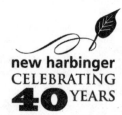

new harbinger
CELEBRATING
40 YEARS